Beautiful Face, Beautiful Body

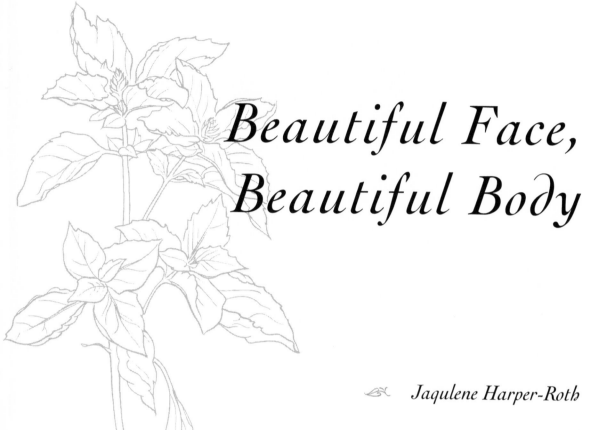

Beautiful Face, Beautiful Body

Jaqulene Harper-Roth

B

Berkley Books • New York

❧ Disclaimer

By using only natural ingredients in their raw, active state, you'll know that the home-made preparations you create from the recipes in this book are nontoxic, hypoallergenic and, of course, fresh. However, all beauty preparations, whether made at home or pur-chased from a shop, should be kept out of the reach of children and pets. Although they may smell delicious enough to eat, these beauty treatments are for external use only, unless otherwise stated. Some natural ingredients are poisonous if consumed, even though it's safe to use them externally. If you have sensitive skin, it is essential to per-form several patch tests to ensure you won't have an allergic reaction to a recipe or ingredient. (See instructions for performing the skin patch test on page 34.) It's possible to have a tolerance to a product or ingredient, but after a few months of trouble-free use, a reaction occurs.

Despite the advice offered here, it is simply impossible to predict an individual's reaction to a particular recipe, remedy, or procedure. Readers should consult a qualified physician or medical caregiver with questions. Neither Berkley Books nor Jaqulene Harper-Roth accepts responsibility for any problems that may arise from use of the fol-lowing recipes.

Acknowledgments

I hope with this book to bring natural beauty back into the home. To you, the reader, I offer the following recipes and remedies to keep your natural beauty for the rest of your life. My aim is to give guidance and tips on skin age prevention with nutrient-replenishing, skin-toning, hair-conditioning, and blemish-clearing natural remedies and simple rituals. I wouldn't be here today without the help, encouragement, and guidance of the following people, who brought this from scribbled notes to a published book.

First, I would like to honor the memory of my grandmother Gladys Lumbard, who guided my experiments with beautifying bathing waters and dusting powders. I must thank all the ladies and gents who generously donated their family recipes for beauty and skin care. I thank my sister Christine for allowing me to experiment with formulas and ingredients for the natural hair dyes in her salon, and the many friends and customers who graciously wore the chameleonlike color changes through weeks of experiments. I am grateful to Candice, Stefanie, and Gustavo, who during the past three years have brought culture, inspiration, happiness, and love, with good old common sense, to my children, especially during those times when Mom was out of bounds, up to her neck in retypes and scribbled notes. I thank my three tots, Zak, Josh, and Tamara, for all the hugs and kisses after long days of researching and writing, not to mention their help with the reams of photocopying.

I thank my husband, Gil, for his faith in my ability to write and complete this book, run an active household, carpool, and raise our children, instilling in them our beliefs of animal equality, vegetarianism, love of life, and natural health. I thank all my cats for sustaining my sanity while I split my time between working and motherhood.

I would like to give a special thank-you to Noah Lukeman, my agent, for his insight and meticulous eye for detail, especially with our American/English punctuation differentials! He had from the start an utter belief in my abilities to become a published author.

I am grateful to my editor, Lisa Considine, for taking a chance with my ideas and experience and for her help in turning a raw manuscript into a book.

Many of the homemade remedies and recipes that follow—the body oils, cleansers, shampoos, intensive conditioners, hair dyes, and scrubs—were donated by ordinary people. The recipes they so generously shared with me have been passed on from generation to generation and use effective techniques and natural ingredients.

✍ *Recipe Contributors*

Sally Allen, Annie Anderson, Annha Anderson, Annha Ash, Queenie Black, Victoria Billington, Molly Briggs, Olive Brown, Shelley Browning, Joanne Causley, Charlie Chambers, John Cox, Susy Day, Tom Enthwhistle, Dilly Farthing, De De Farrow, Christine German, Jo Grant, Sonja Harper, Nigel Hatherley, Reggie Hooks, Patsy Ireland, Pammy Kerr, Gladys Lumbard, Millie Maid, Jennifer Miller, Lori Mills, Millie Oaks, Ed Otterly, Vicky Palfrey, Christine Palmer, Linda Parker, Denise Potter, Jane Potheridge, Petula Prince, Mary Rennolds, Claire Sapford, Trudi Solf, Crystal Sparks, Tina Spiller, Kathleen Stamp, Shannon Taylor, Aaron Thomas, Hannha Thomas, Adriana Vincent, Molly Walters, Patrica Waring, Gabriella Watts, Agnes White, Barbara White, and Sam Wooten.

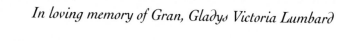

In loving memory of Gran, Gladys Victoria Lumbard

Contents

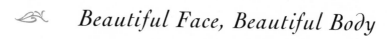 *Beautiful Face, Beautiful Body*

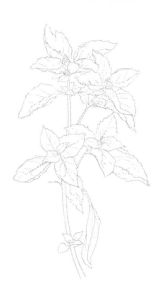

Overview

Natural beauty has played an important role in history since the earliest civilizations when womankind first put plants and other natural elements provided by Mother Earth to use. Formulas for skin softening oils, creams, and lotions date back to biblical times when women rubbed concoctions made from olive oil and spices into their feet to keep them smooth and supple. Scented barks, roots, and rhizomes were finely ground to make body powders. They massaged precious aromatic oils into their hair to keep it smelling sweet. The first lip makeup was made over 5,000 years ago in Egypt. Cleopatra relied on hundreds of natural beauty remedies to maintain her legendary powers of seduction. At that time, facial powders were made from crushed sesame seeds, rice, and barley grains; hair color and tints were made from walnut and henna extracts; eye makeup was made from kohl crayons and crushed semiprecious stones such as malachite and lapis lazuli. Lipsticks of the brightest reds were made from crushed ant eggs and beetles. Many other legendary beauties have attributed their looks (at least in part) to natural beauty secrets.

Modern cosmetology is shrouded in technological mystery, yet the formulas for many beauty remedies are rooted in herbal lore and employ techniques handed down through generations. Making your own health-promoting and beauty preparations is simple, enjoyable, and rewarding. You'll save a great deal of money too! Homemade recipes contain far more active, live ingredients such as essential fatty acids, minerals, vitamins, proteins, and important bioflavonoids than their commercial counterparts. Homemade preparations can be customized to suit individual needs. Soon after you start making your own creations, you'll be hooked.

Recipes offered in this book range from simple blends of body oils, cleansers, and moisturizers to more complex formulas for shampoos, masks, body packs, and hair colors. This book also contains effective treatments (taken internally) for skin disorders such as psoriasis, acne, and eczema. Unlike commercial cosmetics, your own creations spare animals from testing and save your skin from harsh chemicals that ensure prolonged shelf life. Commercial products are made to withstand a wide range of hazards, such as freezing or boiling temperatures, exposure to sunlight, and lengthy storage. Making your own beauty treatments means you'll use them when they're fresh and their ingredients are still fully active. In contrast, commercial products are sometimes shipped halfway around the world to shops and stores where they may sit for up to six months before you, the consumer, use them. The word *natural* is a familiar sight on packaging of commercial cosmetics today, yet there is no accepted standard for its use, so it can mean anything the manufacturer intends it to mean. With your own creations, you'll know they contain only the highest quality ingredients, and you'll know they're fresh.

The following recipes for making natural, living beauty preparations are remarkably simple. You do not need to be a cosmetic scientist or hold a degree in biotechnology to make them. You need only the will, time, and patience. Although you may find some of the smells and textures a little strange at first, all these recipes have been tried and tested, and my family's robust health and glowing skin is living proof that they work.

Most of the ingredients you'll need are already in your pantry, garden, refrigerator, bathroom, and laundry cabinets. It is quite remarkable just how many everyday items you take for granted. Natural cooking oils, cereals, dairy, and fresh produce can all be put to good use on your skin. You can grow herbs, fruit, and vegetables in your garden, or if space is a problem (we don't all have 100 acres to play with), in a window box, rooftop container garden, or kitchen planter. Don't be discouraged if you live in a high-rise apartment. The fresh produce you'll need is only as far as your local supermarket or health food store. And everyone has access to mail-order herbal and natural food suppliers.

If you live on a shoestring, this book is for you. Natural cosmetics are not expensive. The challenge is in balancing the correct ingredients. All the recipes for ageless, beautiful skin, whether applied directly on your skin or consumed for internal cleansing, can be tailor-made to suit your tastes.

Making something for yourself is always more rewarding than buying cosmetics (probably made over a year ago) from a store, especially when you suspect the commercial product has been tested on animals. If you are one whose heart sinks at the thought of all those technicians testing and retesting the latest beauty miracle product, then take heart in what you find between the covers of this book. Be your own guinea pig, learn by all your delicious mistakes, and marvel at the end product. How satisfying to say, "I did this myself. I made something that is good for my whole body, outside in and inside out."

That's how I got started. I had been making skin care recipes for a few years, and I began to wonder how many other people were doing the same thing. It occurred to me that my grandmother's generation just didn't have the money to go out and buy skin beautifying products. I posted notices asking others to share their homemade treatments in local senior citizen centers, churches, coffee shops, and tearooms in and around the counties of Devon and Cornwall, England, where I lived at the time. The response was tremendous, and soon I had recipes for all kinds of skin conditions and beautifying techniques for all walks of life. It took me over a year to work my way through all the recipes, testing to ensure that each actually worked and sometimes searching for substitute ingredients that were easier to find but still did the same job. This book is a combination of those donations and my own tried-and-true recipes.

Being a mother of three small children, I use both my training as a natural healer and common sense in caring for their skin, diet, and overall well-being. I wash their delicate skin in cereal milk, which I immerse in their running bath with natural, sweet-smelling plant extracts that are soothing, cleansing, and relaxing. My daughter, who has very sensitive skin, bathes in chamomile flower infusion and oat milk. I make a wonderful, healing body and diaper powder out of comfrey root, arrowroot, goldenseal, and slippery elm bark. All my children eat a rich diet of natural foods, juices, and micronutrient green shakes. Whenever I look into their happy and healthy faces, I know I am doing the very best for them.

You can do the same thing for yourself and your family. Nature is waiting for you to welcome her into your life. Give these recipes and remedies a try. Your mirror will soon reflect back the beauty that comes from treating yourself with the best nature has to offer.

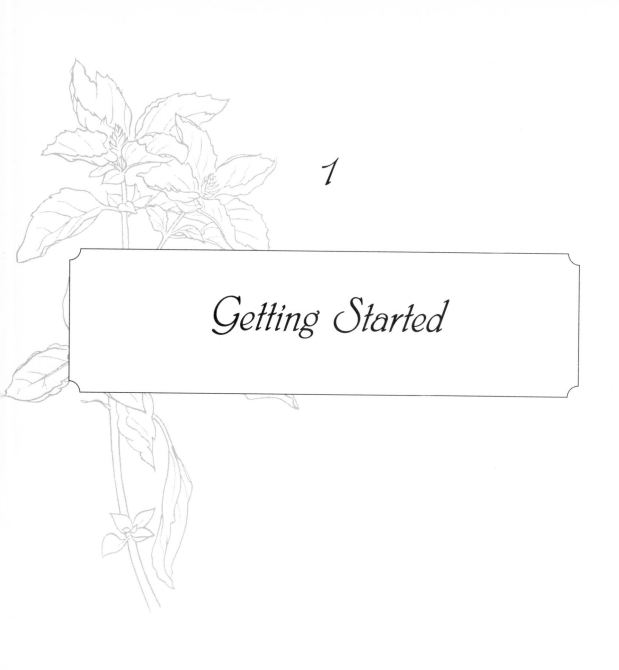

1

Getting Started

Living Ingredients Guide

Natural oils are used as active ingredients for homemade cosmetics because they are skin-nourishing, moisturizing, water-resistant, cell-regenerating, and lubricating. Herb and flower oils are made through methods of cold and heat infusion, steam distillation, bud maceration, and cold-pressing, without the use of harsh chemicals or extreme heat.

Essential oils are the volatile oils extracted from flowers and herbs to make the concentrated, pure essential oils that are used as active ingredients for the recipes in part II. Most essential oils are derived by the steam distillation of fresh herbal plant matter, including leaves, stems, flowers, seeds, and barks. Essential oils are highly concentrated and should always be treated with great care. It takes hundreds of pounds of plant material to produce just one ounce of essential oil. Like the herbs from which the oils are derived, they should be stored carefully. All oils must be diluted before using directly on the skin, as in their raw, highly concentrated state they can burn your skin. They are first mixed with a light vegetable or seed oil, such as sweet almond, grape seed, jojoba bean, olive, or sunflower. Pure essential oils are intended for external use only. They can be fatally poisonous if consumed in sufficient quantity. They are also highly irritating to the mucous membranes of the body and may cause allergic reactions. Clove and cinnamon pure essential oils must be highly diluted as they are known skin irritants.

Essential oil prices are as volatile as the oils themselves. The herbs are harvested from all over the world, and the prices may reflect a costly distillation process, crop abundance or failure, or soil quality. As beauty aids, essential oils are useful in caring for the whole body. They are multifunctional, working as skin rejuvenators, vitality enhancers, and health remedies. Various oils can soothe, relax, or excite as they penetrate the dermal skin layers. For instance, the essential oil of lavender helps to balance sebum production and therefore is an excellent treatment for acne and dry skin conditions, as well as for an anxious mind. All essential oils are naturally antiseptic, and many have antibacterial, antifungal, and antiviral properties. What follows is a list of oils most commonly used in natural beauty preparations. It is not necessary to purchase them all at once. Start with two or three, enough to prepare a few recipes that appeal to you or address a particular concern. It's often more economical to buy these essential oils from herbal suppliers or aromatherapy outlets, which customarily sell these oils in 1–1½ ounce dropper bottles. If secured tightly after each use, one bottle will last for years.

OIL	USED IN
Basil	Massage oils, baths, facial steams, hair care, oral hygiene
Bergamot	Antiagers, hand and foot care, massage oils, scrubs and packs
Carrot seed	Massage, skin care, antiagers, hair care
Clary sage	Foot care, oral hygiene, hair care, exotic baths, body packs
Cypress	Swollen vein soaks and rubs, massage oils, antiagers
Fennel	Eye care, soothing skin creams, shampoos, perfumes, teeth
Frankincense	Sensual massage, antiagers, skin care, baths
Geranium	Hair care, massage, antiagers, baths, moisturizers

Ginger	Massage oils, antiagers, hair care, baths
Jasmine	Skin care, massage oils, baths, moisturizers
Juniper berry	Hair care, massage oils, antiagers
Lavender	Perfumes, hair care, massage, skin care, steams
Lemon	Antiagers, skin care, hand and foot treatments, massage, hair
Lemon balm (melissa)	Hair care, facial steams, skin care, massage oils
Mandarin	Antiagers, facial cleansers, masks, scrubs, moisturizers
Myrrh	Skin care, antiagers, baths, massage oils
Neroli (orange blossom)	Moisturizers, baths, skin care, massage oils, antiagers
Peppermint	Hair care, oral hygiene, massage oils, baths, facial tonics
Pine	Body packs, hair care, massage oils
Rose	Sensual massage oils, moisturizers, foot and hand care
Rosemary	Hair care, massage oils, skin care, baths
Rosewood	Sensual massage oils, exotic baths, skin care
Sandalwood	Facial steams, massage oils, antiagers, skin care
Sweet marjoram	Massage oils, skin care, hair care, baths
Tea tree	Natural antiseptic, temple massage oils, facial cleansers, steams
Thyme, sweet	Hair and scalp care, exotic baths, massage oils
Ylang ylang	Hair care, exotic baths, sensual massage oils, antiagers

PURE ESSENTIAL OILS TO *AVOID* DURING PREGNANCY

Aniseed	Cedarwood	Cypress
Basil	Cinnamon	Hyssop
Bay	Coriander	Juniper berry

Lemongrass
Marjoram
Myrrh
Nutmeg

Pennyroyal
Peppermint
Rosemary
Savory

Tansy
Wintergreen

PURE ESSENTIAL OILS *RECOMMENDED* DURING PREGNANCY

Bergamot
Catnip
Chamomile
Citrus oils
Clary sage

Geranium
Jasmine
Lavender
Melissa
Neroli

Rose
Spearmint
Ylang ylang

RELAXING ESSENTIAL OILS

Chamomile
Geranium

Lavender
Petigrain

Rose

ENERGIZING ESSENTIAL OILS

Cypress
Juniper berry
Lime

Patchouli
Peppermint
Rosemary

Rosewood
Tangerine

ANTISEPTIC AND HEALING ESSENTIAL OILS

Calendula
Eucalyptus

Lavender
Peppermint

Tea tree
Wintergreen

Aniseed	Clove	Thuja
Bitter almond	Hyssop	Wintergreen
Cinnamon	Sage	

Note that sage pure oil can be toxic, even in the most minute amounts. It should never be used by pregnant and lactating women or children and should not be used on the skin. For an herb that functions like sage but without the toxic side effects, use clary sage.

Cold-Pressed Plant Oils

The following plant oils are cold-pressed. Delicate live extracts derived from the raw plant matter can be destroyed through high heat or chemical extraction. Cold-pressing oils preserves those sensitive ingredients. While these oils are more expensive than refined oils, they are also free of the petroleum residues used in the refining process. Using cold-pressed plant oils in natural beauty preparations is better for the environment and your precious, delicate skin.

Apricot kernel oil	Jojoba bean oil
Avocado oil	Palm kernel oil
Castor oil	Sesame seed oil
Coconut oil	Sweet almond oil
Corn oil	Sunflower seed oil
Grape seed oil	Virgin olive oil
Ground nut oil	Walnut oil
Hazelnut oil	Wheat germ (berry) oil

Herbs can be used in either fresh or dried form. When collecting and harvesting fresh herbs from your garden or the open countryside, you'll need a brown paper bag and an illustrated botanical dictionary. Even if you think you know what you are looking for, why risk harvesting a possibly toxic look-alike? You need a pocket-sized book that has detailed, colored diagrams showing flower parts, bark textures, root formations, and aerial parts, with descriptions of the plant's natural habitat. *Wildflower Folklore* by Laura C. Martin and *Dictionary of Plant Names* by Allen J. Coombes are two good ones.

Collect only young, firm plants, and be careful not to damage the whole plant if you need only a part. If you need only a few flower petals, cut them off. Don't tear, twist, or rip off plant parts, then leave the poor thing to die. Put what you need in the paper bag and leave the rest of the plant unharmed. Always remember when out foraging in the open countryside that all plants are part of an interwoven, intricate habitat balanced by Mother Nature for the needs and survival of many wild animals, birds, and insects. As a visitor to their home, respect the laws of nature.

Harvest herbs after the morning dew has dried or in the early evening when the sun goes down. When you get home, carefully wash your harvest except for the delicate flower petals. Check petals for insects (you don't want any insect eggs and tiny beetles in your lotion) and damaged parts, but don't wash them. Carefully lay the clean herbs to dry on a mesh drying rack or some folded paper towels in a warm, dark, well-ventilated place until you need them. It is better to use the herbs you've collected right away, but this is not always convenient or practical. Good quality dried herbs still retain much of their potency and life force.

To dry harvested herbs and flowers, hang them in small bundles in a warm, well-ventilated room, place them on a wire mesh drying rack, or dry them in a brown paper bag. Make sure the plants are kept out of direct sunlight. Keep out of the reach of curious children and pets. If you dry your herbs in paper bags, make sure that you label and date the contents with the common and Latin name, and note where it was picked for future reference.

If you have the space and time, collecting, drying, and cultivating garden or wild herbs can be half the fun. Even children can take part. It makes the whole exercise from beginning to end more rewarding. Since this is not always possible or practical, there are many herbal suppliers that use organic farming methods and do most of the basic preparation for you. (See the appendix for mail-order sources). Whatever your herb source, make sure that the plant is brightly colored with a fresh, pungent aroma and as whole as possible. Powdered herbs lose a lot of their potency during the grinding and packaging process. When you receive herbs through the mail, smell them. If they lack a fresh scent or smell of chemicals or mold, send them back. Whenever possible, buy your herbs from suppliers that use organic farming methods and wild-crafted techniques.

Camomile or Chamomile Flowers   Freshly harvested, these delicate, sweet-apple-scented, daisylike flowers are grown by the acre in Europe for their essential oil. Many of the recipes and remedies in this book call for chamomile (as an infusion or essential oil) because it is so gentle, relaxing, sweet-smelling, and soothing to the skin and spirit. Chamomiles come in several different varieties, but unless otherwise specified, the recipes in this book concentrate on the German (*Matricaria chamomilla*) type. Chamomile is cooling and nonirritating. It is a vasoconstrictor, shrinking small blood vessels and reducing redness in the cheeks. Chamomile is one of the few oils traditionally used for children's and babies' delicate skin. In combination with lavender, chamomile essential oil diluted in water makes an excellent, refreshing facial and body splash.

Comfrey   Dried roots and leaves of the comfrey plant are used in cosmetic preparations as it possesses a remarkable ability to bind broken tissues and stimulate new growth. I regularly use its finely ground roots in a soothing baby powder. It is especially soothing for diaper rash as it heals open, sometimes bleeding, sore bottoms. Use this often overlooked wild weed for bathing recipes, facials, body mists, and soothing skin creams.

Dandelion   Fresh dandelion flowers and leaves are very nutritious, but I also put them to work in homemade cosmetics. I have used the flowers, stems (and milk), leaves, and roots. Not one bit of this remarkable weed goes to waste. Dandelion is an excellent ingredient for soothing skin salves, aiding the regeneration of skin in those who suffer from eczema and psoriasis. It is used in misting tonics and antiaging lotions to bleach age spots and freckles. The white, sticky fluid inside the stem, known in English folklore as milky dashel juice, is widely used as an herbal remedy for treating warts.

Eucalyptus   There are approximately 300 varieties of this herb, all with powerful antibacterial and antiviral properties. I use it in the bath, either as drops of essential oil or a warm infusion of the fresh leaves. Eucalyptus has healing properties that are effective on congested or septic skin. It limits excess sebum production, and in its essential oil form, it can be applied neat with a cotton bud on pimples. Eucalyptus is also a tissue regenerator; it has mild estrogenic properties and, like aloe, helps heal burns.

Fennel   Dried fennel seeds and essential oil are frequently used as ingredients for eye gels, moisturizers, perfumes, and shampoos. I have also found it to be a pleasant-tasting addition to mouthwashes and toothpastes. Its subtle, soothing aroma makes it a good ingredient for body and foot powders. Fennel is a wonderful natural remedy in the form of an herbal tea, ideal for calming motion and morning sickness, and it can even increase the production of milk in nursing mothers. Fennel essential oil is an antiwrinkle aid that balances sebum production. **Caution:** Never use fennel essential oil on children or people suffering with epilepsy. The powerful oil penetrates the skin and can cause convulsions.

Geranium (Rose Geranium)   Freshly harvested and dried leaves, as well as the essential oil, are all fragrance enhancers for moisturizers and facial lotions, inducing a sense of inner well-being and restful sleep. Geranium essential oil acts to balance most complexions, cleansing and refreshing. It is strongly astringent and a known lymphatic stimulator, releasing fluid from water-saturated complexions. Geranium in the form of an herbal infusion is used in nighttime moisturizers, body oils, and sensual massaging lotions.

Ginseng   This root is an excellent skin conditioner and cleanser. It has tonic and stimulating effects on the skin. I have used it in conjunction with herbs, such as chamomile, dandelion, and horsetail, for skin-nutritious splashes and baths.

Lavender   This versatile and honored herb is calming, soothing, and balancing. The essential oil can be applied undiluted to burns and pimples and is known to increase the rate of healing. It balances sebum production, reduces scarring, and inhibits bacterial growth. Freshly harvested or dried leaves and flowers are used in many bathing tonics, hair refreshers, and skin-nourishing mists. Use the essential oil in moisturizers, massage oils, sunburn healing lotions, and insect-bite soothing creams.

Lemon Balm (Melissa)   Lemon balm flowers, leaves, and the essential oil are potent ingredients in natural insect repellents and treatments for poison ivy. Lemon balm bathing infusions and body mists make your skin tingle. The essential oil is rare and extremely expensive. Use it in a dilution of 1 percent, or you will end up intensifying the conditions you are trying to alleviate. You'll need only two to four drops in a full tub for bathing.

Marigold (Calendula)   Don't confuse this herb with Tagetes (or African marigold), which is often planted in flower beds and vegetable gardens as a natural insect repellent. Tagetes marigold is neither edible nor medicinal. For the recipes in this book, you'll need pot marigold (or *Calendula officinalis*). The petals, fresh juice, and essential oil are all used in hair care treatments, color-enhancing pastes and rinses, antiseptic creams, body oils, and facial toners. This herb has remarkable healing properties. An active antiseptic and bacteria fighter, it's used in many skin-healing aids.

Mint   Fresh and dried mint leaves and flowers are both edible and medicinal. Of the three main varieties (there are over thirty hybrid species) used in cosmetics, peppermint, spearmint, and catnip essential oils are the most potent. Peppermint is used in oral hygiene and hair care preparations. I put spearmint in natural toothpastes, headache-relieving lotions, and foot care creams. Catnip is generally mixed with other healing herbs for baby care preparations. Catnip tea is very soothing to babies suffering with infant colic. Cats, of course, love it!

Myrrh   This naturally occurring resin has a pungent, spicy aroma. It is an anti-inflammatory agent and can rejuvenate mature, wrinkled skin. Myrrh in the form of a tincture is used in antiaging skin creams and indulgent bathing rituals.

Plantain   Used fresh in herbal first aid, plantain cools burns. The dried roots, leaves, and flowers all make soothing skin salves, burn creams, and infusion baths.

Rose   Freshly picked rose petals sprinkled in an evening bath utterly enchant a deflated spirit. The soft, feminine fragrance of the essential oil makes it a natural choice for skin care and massage recipes. Rose is used as an active ingredient in toilet waters, facial and hair steams, and some baby care treatments. The aromatic water (a by-product of the essential oil processing) can be used as a skin toner. Its soothing, antiseptic properties are suitable for all skin types, especially mature and overly dry complexions. Rose essential oil is extremely expensive, as much as $800 to $1,000 an ounce. An anti-inflammatory and astringent, it tones the capillaries, which lay just beneath the skin's surface. Pregnant women should avoid using the essential oil, which is absorbed through the skin and the bloodstream, as its properties can be overpowering. It's been known to cause premature uterine contractions.

Sage   Freshly harvested or dried leaves and flowers are familiar ingredients in natural cosmetics. Both help balance excess fluid and clear congested skin layers. Sage essential oil, on the other hand, can be toxic even in the most minute quantities and is believed to cause uterine spasms, so it should be avoided by pregnant women. Instead, use clary sage, an essential oil with properties akin to fresh and dried sage.

Sandalwood   A soothing, aromatic herb with powerful antibacterial properties, sandalwood is uplifting and energizing. It is an excellent ingredient for massage oils, moisturizing lotions, and bathing recipes.

Tea Tree (Melaneuca alternifolia)   Tea tree essential oil, an antiseptic, preservative, immune stimulant, wound binder, infection fighter, acne combatant, and skin soother, is one of nature's greatest healers. Tea tree essential oil should be a part of all earth-wise first aid kits. It is nontoxic and preserves healthy tissue while reducing the risk of scars.

Thyme (Thymus vulgaris linalol or Sweet Thyme)   The essential oil of sweet thyme is safe to use in skin preparations, but avoid oils of other varieties of thyme, which are known to be extremely toxic. In a dilution of pure water, this essential oil is reputed for its treatment of hair loss and is in many other natural cosmetics to suppress the growth of microorganisms.

Violet   These pretty, delicate, pungent flowers have been used for centuries for soothing mouthwashes and toilet waters. The freshly picked flower petals are edible. Freshly harvested leaves are used in remedies for menstrual water retention, nervous headaches, ear infections, sinus fevers, whooping cough, flu, pleurisy, and tonsillitis. Violets are multifunctional garden herbs. They are nutritious, skin-enhancing, and they make a wonderful posy for Mother's Day.

Witch Hazel   Dried witch hazel bark and leaves, or if you have them growing in your garden, freshly harvested leaves, can be used for skin care in soothing gels and balms, pore-tightening tonics, and gentle facial masks. Natural toothpastes and mouthwashes often contain witch hazel.

Yarrow   Fresh or dried yarrow is used as an active ingredient in homemade skin care moisturizers and hair-loss tonics. It has excellent cleansing and astringent qualities and can be used in the form of a cooled infusion for a natural douche.

Ylang Ylang   Traditionally used for its properties as an aphrodisiac, ylang ylang has a sweet, heavy, pungent aroma. The essential oil is generally mixed with a lighter citrus oil, such as bergamot or tangerine, to balance its pungency, and the combinations make wonderful, sensual massage oils. A few drops of the essential oil can be applied directly on the skin to balance oily complexions.

Fruits, Vegetables, and Wild Edibles

Wild edibles and fruits and vegetables from gardens have been harvested as healing and skin care agents for centuries. I've experimented extensively with those listed below. All contain active, living micronutrients that digest surface bacteria, unclog congested pores, and leave your complexion glowing.

You should harvest wild edibles such as seasonal berries and leaves with respect for their natural habitats. Always take an illustrated botanical dictionary with you. There are several good guides available, but I recommend *Dictionary of Plant Names* by Allen J. Coombes and *Peterson Field Guide to Edible Wild Plants*.

When buying fresh produce, try to buy organic. You don't want to put pesticides and fertilizers on your skin. Additionally, produce left to ripen in the sun (as much organic produce is) is more potent than produce left to ripen in boxes. Many nonorganic root vegetables are waxed to preserve them, so they might be anywhere from six months to two years old. For use in the recipes in this book, these waxed skins and peels must be removed, and with them go the valuable micronutrients embedded in them. Organic produce doesn't look bright and glossy, but the goodness is there, on the inside. Organic produce is sweeter and packed with more active vitamins, minerals, and enzymes.

The first rule in using produce is that it must be fresh, as well as free of bruises and blemishes. It should show no signs of decomposition. If it's not fit to eat, it's not fit to be used in my recipes, either. Thoroughly wash and air-dry your harvest, then refrigerate whatever you're not going to use right away in an airtight plastic or glass container.

Apples (all varieties)	Dandelions	Melons
Apricots	Dill (flowers and	Onions
Avocados	seeds)	Orange
Bananas	Fennel	Parsley
Blackberries	Figs	Peaches
Broccoli	Grapes	Pears
Cabbage (white and	Kiwifruit	Plums
purple)	Lemons	Rose hips
Carrots	Lettuce (all varieties)	Strawberries
Cherries	Mangoes	Tomatoes
Cucumber	Marigold (flowers)	

The following is a list of ingredients that you'll be using to make your homemade cosmetics. You'll find most in your kitchen, around your home, or in your local supermarket, pharmacy, or health food store. You are probably already using many of these daily in one form or another. I really enjoy browsing through the aisles of health food and specialty stores, where the assistants are more than willing to help me find what I need and are often intrigued by my projects. If you are unsure about an item, ask. You may have to order some supplies by mail. These companies usually have a wealth of information, so either write or telephone for more details.

Aloe Vera   Aloe has been used as a skin treatment since the times of Cleopatra. It is a remarkable healer and internal cleanser. A member of the lily family, it has succulent green leaves that produce a thick, clear gel. Aloe gel is made from the plant's natural juice, which is 99 percent water. The remaining 1 percent contains well over twenty different amino acids and carbohydrates. Aloe possesses skin-rejuvenating qualities and aids the healing of burns.

Apple Cider Vinegar   All vinegars are known for their high acid content. In cosmetic preparations, apple cider vinegar is used to remove alkaline residues from the skin and scalp. It should always be applied in a diluted form (1 part vinegar, 8 parts water). Apple cider vinegar is frequently used in skin-toning astringents, refreshing body mists, and hair rinses. It restores the correct pH balance of the skin and gives a rich, glossy shine to hair. It tightens hair cuticles, increases luster, and improves manageability. A very weak solution of cider vinegar and water makes an excellent vaginal douche and shallow bath for the treatment of yeast infections.

Arnica Tincture   Arnica tincture is an efficient skin soother used for drawing out bruises. Made from the dried flowers of the arnica plant, this tincture has been used for centuries by homeopathic practitioners for treating sore, swollen skin. Cleansers and gels with arnica tincture help to reduce puffiness.

Arrowroot   An edible starch, arrowroot is used as a thickener for moisturizers, creams, and lotions. It is an excellent emulsifier and absorbent and is often used as the basic ingredient for soothing powders for the body and feet.

Baking Soda   This is a white powder prepared by treating soda ash (sodium carbonate) with carbon dioxide. It adds a smooth texture to creams and lotions. Baking soda adjusts the skin's pH and stabilizes viscosity. It is nontoxic and traditionally used in effervescent bathing treatments, toothpastes, and mouthwashes. It makes an excellent addition to natural deodorants and body powders.

Beeswax   A natural wax produced by bees, it is added to creams, moisturizers, balms, and lotions primarily as an emulsifier. It is nontoxic and possesses natural germ-killing properties. In natural, living cosmetics, it forms a protective barrier on the skin's surface, guarding against irritants and locking in precious moisture.

Benzoin Resin   Native to Southeast Asia, this mild, natural preservative has limited use in treatments. Benzoin has a spicy and heady aroma. It relieves irritation, itching, redness, and cracking of the skin. When you're shopping for it, make sure that the resin has been diluted in wood alcohol, not ethyol glycol.

Borax   A white powder that consists of alkaline crystals made from a natural mineral, borax is commonly used in industry as a water softener. Borax acts as a natural antiseptic, although it should never be used directly on the skin or an open wound. You'll see borax listed as an ingredient in many natural commercial products such as shampoos and soaps.

Brewer's Yeast   Brewer's yeast is an active ingredient in facial masks, especially anti-aging formulas, due to its deep cleansing action and excellent nourishing properties. It makes a refreshing eye treat when combined with fresh juices or buttermilk.

Burdock Root   Burdock root is used in baths and facial steams to cleanse the skin and purify the sweat glands of toxic waste accumulations. It restores skin tone and smoothness, heals irritations, and promotes cell regeneration. Burdock root infusion or tincture is used in many of my facial and skin washes.

Buttermilk   Much like other dairy products, buttermilk is used as an ingredient for natural cosmetics. It is very soothing to the skin's surface and especially soothing to tired, heavy eyes.

Calamine Lotion   Made from the rhizome of the sweet flag plant, calamine lotion is 95 percent zinc oxide and 5 percent iron oxide, which gives its characteristic pink color. As it dries on the skin, this liquid cools sore sunburn. Its properties are put to work in skin tonics and facial washes.

Carotene   Carotene is a precursor of vitamin A, and it occurs naturally in plants (especially yellow and orange vegetables), algae, and butter. In cosmetics, carotene is used as coloring. It prevents oxidation and is nontoxic.

Chlorophyll   The green life force of plants is essential to photosynthesis. It is a microcrystalline wax used in natural toothpastes, creams, and deodorants. Like carotene, it is sometimes used as coloring.

Cocoa Butter   A solid fat obtained by roasting seeds of *Theobroma cacao*, cocoa butter is used as an emollient. Cocoa butter melts at body temperature and is used in skin care during pregnancy, helping to prevent stretch marks.

Corn Flour/Cornstarch   This highly absorbent ingredient is found in many natural face and body powders, baby care products (especially diaper rash creams and powders), and a few dry shampoo recipes. Both cornstarch and corn flour are fine, white powders made from corn kernels. Both have natural healing properties that soothe the skin's surface.

Folic Acid   A member of the vitamin B complex, folic acid is used as an emollient and scalp treatment to thicken hair strands.

Fuller's Earth   This finely powdered ingredient looks like clay. It is mined from reclaimed areas of the seabed. You can generally purchase white or brown varieties in one-ounce quantities. Fuller's earth is used in body masks and scrubs due to its highly absorbent properties.

Glycerin   A by-product of soap manufacturing, glycerin is a humectant and mild emulsifier. It's used in natural cosmetics to hold moisture, keeping preparations from drying out. It is odorless, colorless, and tacky.

Honey   A natural mixture of 98 percent raw sugars and 2 percent active micronutrients, honey has mild antiseptic properties, which prevent bacterial growth. It is added to moisturizers, hand creams, facial cleansers, and many body lotions. In the raw, natural state, honeys (clear, solid, floral, or herbal) are very nutritious to eat.

Kaolin (China Clay)   This pure clay originated from the Kaolin Hill in the Kiangsi Province of eastern China. It is used in many beauty preparations, sometimes as a substitute for fuller's earth. It creates subtle hair highlights and is also used in body powders, deep-cleansing masks, and facial packs. Bentonite clay, mined in the Midwest and Canada, can be substituted for kaolin.

Kelp   A rich mucilage and gelling agent, kelp contains many marine minerals and active vitamins. It makes an excellent ingredient for facial masks and deep-cleansing body packs because it is very skin-nourishing and absorbent. I make a weekly seaweed body pack to soothe and heal irritated psoriasis lesions during stressful flare-ups.

Lanolin   This wax is produced by the oil glands of sheep. No harm comes to the animal, because lanolin is separated from the wool. Lanolin is easily absorbed by the skin, making it an excellent moisturizer. Anhydrous lanolin, which is protective and water soluble, is prepared by reducing lanolin's natural water content. It is claimed that lanolin has greater penetrating power than petroleum or beeswax because its composition and molecular structure is nearly identical to the lipids in human skin.

Lecithin   Lecithin is a waxy oil, usually derived from eggs or soybeans, though it is present in all living cells. It is a commonly used antioxidant and an emulsifier in lotions and creams.

Maple Syrup A natural resource of raw, active sugars, maple syrup comes from the sap of the Canadian *Acer saccharum* tree. It has moisturizing and slightly antiseptic qualities and is often used as a substitute for honey.

Oatmeal/Oat Bran Soothing and healing to the skin's surface, oatmeal and oat bran gently exfoliate dead skin cells and unclog the pores of impurities. Oats are a perfect ingredient for treating overly dry complexions, irritated, blemished, or sensitive skin. In combination with slippery elm bark, oatmeal makes a soothing and cleansing bath for children suffering from chicken pox. The thick paste is applied over the oozing pustules. The dry paste forms a hard crust, virtually impossible to scratch off. Both oatmeal and oat bran are included in many facial scrubs and cleansers.

Orrisroot Orrisroot is a fragrant rhizome that has become an important perfume fixative. It can take up to six years to harvest (four years to grow, two years to dry). For this reason alone, it is very expensive. Ground into a fine powder, orrisroot is included in many natural body powders and dry-hair shampoos.

Papain This enzyme, found in papaya fruit, is used widely in exfoliants. It smooths the skin by dissolving dead skin cells.

Paraffin Paraffin is a translucent white wax made from petroleum and is used to thicken creams, lotions, lip preparations, and other makeup bases. Paraffin seals the skin, preventing moisture evaporation.

Pectin Pectin is a carbohydrate extracted from apples or citrus fruit. It is used to thicken creams, lotions, and gels. Used externally, it soothes irritated skin; as an internal treatment, it alleviates intestinal discomfort.

Propolis Propolis is a brown gumlike substance that bees make by collecting the sap from tree buds, which they mix with their own secretions. Worker bees generously paint the hive to protect it from bacterial and microbial infestations. Propolis is a strong antiseptic, repels fungal infestations, and has mild painkilling properties. It can be purchased as a thick gum substance, powdered, or in capsules. Propolis is used as a skin protector and is especially soothing in lip balms and healing salves.

Pumice   This lightweight volcanic rock is used for cleansing and sloughing off dead skin. In powdered form, pumice is used in body scrubs and abrasive soaps.

Rhassoul Mud   This fine, powdered clay originates from the Atlas Mountains of Morocco. Rhassoul mud can be purchased from herbal suppliers in one-ounce quantities. It is a deep-cleaning, gritty substance that effectively exfoliates the skin.

Rose Hips   The fruit of the rosebush, rose hips are both tonic and astringent. Rose hips are the richest source of vitamin C when ingested as an herbal tea, juice, or unsweetened fruit jelly. As a natural cosmetic ingredient, rose hips are soothing to irritated and blemished skin.

Royal Jelly   A highly nutritious secretion of worker bees consisting of 31 percent protein, 15 percent carbohydrate, 15 percent vitamins and minerals, royal jelly is powerful stuff! It is one of the most difficult foods to harvest, as it is stored deep within the beehive to feed the queen bee. Although it has been shown to possess miraculous rejuvenating properties, its reputation as an antiager is still in dispute. In natural cosmetics, royal jelly is used in skin-nourishing facial packs and moisturizers.

Shea Butter   Also known as karite butter, shea butter is a vegetable fat from the karite tree, used in cosmetics because it forms a breathable, water-resistant film. Shea butter is nontoxic and used in moisturizers and sunscreens.

Water   Water is a vital component in making natural cosmetics. It is the base for most creams, lotions, shampoos, conditioners, hair dyes, and moisturizers. In fact, I don't think there is a recipe that doesn't use water either as an ingredient or in its application. The water you use as an ingredient for your recipes should be the same quality of filtered, mineral, or spring water that you drink.

Yogurt   A valuable source of amino acids and proteins, yogurt is easily absorbed and makes a soothing, refreshing facial cleanser. It is made by fermenting milk with friendly, health-enhancing bacteria. It is high in calcium and active, predigested vitamins. As a cosmetic ingredient, yogurt balances skin pH and makes an excellent mask for oily complexions.

Zinc Oxide   A skin protectant with the greatest UV (ultraviolet) absorption of all commercial pigments, zinc oxide is used in sunscreens, as an antiseptic, and as an astringent. You'll see it listed as an ingredient in baby care products, especially diaper rash creams and ointments, because of its remarkable tissue-healing and water-resistant qualities.

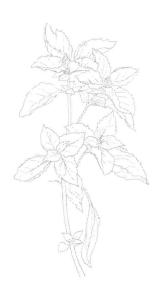

Getting to Work

The great thing about making your own cosmetics is that you already have most of the equipment you'll need in your home. Things you use everyday can lend themselves to your beauty needs, too. I have always had great fun preparing and experimenting with herbal beauty treatments. You don't have to be a great cook to achieve great results in your beauty playground. Cooking is not a passion of mine, but I like to put our pots and pans to equally good use.

I suggest you reserve special equipment solely for natural beauty recipes. Plastic pitchers, spoons, blenders, spatulas, and measuring bowls often absorb and retain both colors and odors. Glass and stainless steel are easier to clean and sterilize. Remember, this equipment needn't be new when you begin experimenting with the following recipes.

Basic Equipment

Accurate Scales Tabletop or diet scales that accurately measure quantities as small as ¼ ounce are the best. When you begin making your cosmetics, exact dry weights are essential, but as you gain more confidence, you will be able to judge by sight how much powder, granules, or grains you require. You'll always need the scales for roots, rhizomes, barks, and heavier herbs. If you are buying your herbs by the ounce, scales may be unnecessary.

Blender   If possible, use a blender with a glass pitcher as they're so much easier to clean and sterilize, and they are less likely to harbor pungent aromas, stains, and residues. I purchased my faithful blender from a yard sale. I use it for grinding nuts and seeds into textured meal as well as whipping air into moisturizers, creams, and oils.

Ceramic Bowls   Ceramic bowls are ideal to use for heating oils and balms. It's best to have a few large and small bowls. When a recipe calls for a small amount of oil or wax to be heated, I place a small ceramic bowl inside a saucepan of warm water (instead of using my double boiler) and mix the other ingredients right in.

Cheesecloth or Mesh Strainers   Both cheesecloth and mesh strainers are used for straining herbs from liquids. Cheesecloth (or panty hose) makes ideal bathing and infusion bags.

Chopping Board   Your chopping board should preferably be made from something other than wood. Wooden chopping boards have a tendency to harbor germs, and they stain easily. The best kind are dishwasher-safe and aren't damaged by heavy use. A marble slab is my first choice, but they are rather expensive. Any Formica or polyethylene board will do.

Coffee Bean or Nut Grinder   I use a small coffee grinder for chopping hard berries and dried roots. It's perfect for grinding the small quantities of nut meals that I use in scrubs. Make sure that your grinder can be dismantled for easy cleaning.

Double Boiler   Double boilers produce a gentle, even heat that is good for blending massage oils, eye gels, balms, salves, and moisturizers. For cosmetic recipes, use one made from stainless steel, glass, or enamel. Teflon and other metals, such as aluminum, cast iron, or copper, will have adverse chemical effects on your recipe outcome.

Funnels   Heat-resistant plastic or stainless steel funnels are invaluable for filling bottles and jars with your finished products. If you have problems finding wide-mouthed funnels, as I have, you can easily make your own from gallon or half gallon plastic milk containers or plastic soda bottles. Simply cut them in half and use the end with the pouring spout.

Glass or Stainless Steel Mixing Bowls   Stick to glass or stainless steel bowls because wood, plastic, and china either stain, chip, or harbor germs.

Grater   A grater is ideal for breaking up soap and vegetable pulp into tiny particles before heating. Plastic and metal graters work equally well.

Measuring Spoons and Cups   In many recipes, exact quantities will ensure a successful result. Use measuring equipment made of stainless steel, glass, or heat-resistant plastic.

Paring Knives   Paring knives are ideal for cutting flowers, herbs, and fruit. They are also good for cutting slithers from blocks of beeswax, soap, cocoa, and shea butter.

Pipette or Eyedropper   A pipette or an eyedropper are useful for measuring minute quantities of resins, infused oils, essential oils, fragrance oils, tinctures, and decoctions.

Pyrex Measuring Cups   Keep on hand small, medium, and large measuring cups to measure liquids such as infusions and water. You'll also find them useful in applying hair treatments and whole-body treatments.

Spatula   Spatulas are ideal for scooping out salves, creams, and lotions from mixing bowls. They are also useful for applying pastes and masks.

Stainless Steel or Enamel Saucepans   Use saucepans for boiling, steaming, and making decoctions (a method to extract the soluble contents of an herb, root, bark, seeds, or berries and transfer it into the water by boiling both ingredients together). Two saucepans can also be used together as a makeshift double boiler.

Surgical Gloves   Latex gloves protect your hands from agents that can stain your skin, such as natural hair dyes, masks, and conditioners. Use them when applying and mixing these products. Cleaning gloves offer terrific protection to your hands but make it hard to handle anything delicate, so it's worth investing in surgical gloves.

Whisk   A small hand whisk is ideal for whipping small quantities of creams, moisturizers, and balms.

🖎 *Storage*

The living beauty recipes and remedies in this book produce relatively small quantities. The idea is to avoid spoilage and subsequent waste. When you do store your beauty recipes in the refrigerator, keep them well away from food you plan to eat. Either place them in an otherwise empty salad compartment or a small cardboard box in the bottom of the refrigerator. Clearly label your products with the name and date of preparation. Store skin care remedies in bathroom cabinets, high out of the reach of curious children and out of direct sunlight. A small circle of waxed paper cut to the size of the jar lid and placed over the cream or lotion before sealing will keep out microscopic life. Add a few drops of lavender, tea tree, or pure wheat germ oil to prevent spoilage. All three are natural preservatives and have been added to beauty treatments for centuries.

Since bacteria love to breed in moist, warm conditions, it is essential that all your storage containers and their lids are kept sterilized and dry. When you have finished with a recipe, wash all your equipment and store it until you need it for another recipe. Store your concoctions in either dark-colored glass or opaque plastic containers with a lid, away from heat, dampness, and sunlight.

A Note About Recycling   Although recycling is admirable, make sure that plastic or glass containers you plan to reuse are cleaned, sterilized, and thoroughly dried. If you do not have a dishwasher, soak containers in hot, soapy water for about ten minutes. Then thoroughly scrub, rinse with hot water, and air-dry. I do not recommend storing beauty preparations in recycled medicine, poison, fertilizer, or household detergent (other than dish washing liquid) bottles.

Bottles   Your can use four-ounce, six-ounce, eight-ounce, ten-ounce, twelve-ounce, and sixteen-ounce plastic or glass bottles. Any liquid can be stored in bottles: infusions, massage oils, shampoos, conditioners, toners, and mouthwashes. I prefer colored glass storage bottles. Dark glass helps preserve the volatile extracts in oil blends.

Brown Paper Bags   Brown paper bags are ideal for holding freshly picked herbs and flowers. I recycle my brown paper grocery bags and use them to dry bulk herbs and roots. I also use the strong brown paper securely screwed under jar lids to keep my dried herbs moisture-free.

Cotton Kitchen Towels   Cotton towels are ideal for covering herbal infusions and mopping up spills. I prefer to use them because paper towels create unnecessary waste.

Large Plastic Container with Tightly Fitting Lid   Store leftover preparations in plastic containers. Make sure that each container is labeled, and store it in a cool, dark place.

Lidded Jars   You can use plastic or colored glass jars. Being a mother of three small children, I recycle baby food jars, which are just the right size for storing creams and salves. You can paint the outside of the glass with brown or blue India ink, opaque it with poster paint, or cover the glass with self-adhesive labels to block out the light completely.

Plastic Wrap   Use plastic wrap to cover preparations that will not be applied immediately. Hair dyes, conditioners, and shampoos can be transferred to a bowl and covered with plastic wrap until you're ready to use them.

Reusable or Self-Sealing Tea Bags   Small, medium, and large reusable tea bags are ideal for mixtures of dry herbs. Fill with sleep-inducing herbs and tuck them inside pillows and eye rests. If you plan to immerse an herb mixture, for a bath, use stainless steel or plastic tea balls.

Shaker Jars   Glass, stainless steel, or plastic shaker jars are ideal for storing herbal body powders, dry shampoos, and facial and body scrubs. These jars are generally used for baking, cake decorating, and spice holders. They can easily lend themselves to your beauty remedies.

Pump Spray Bottles   Spritzer bottles are good for applying body mists, astringents, shower splashes, and toners. Save your room deodorizing and hair spray bottles for this purpose. Wash them thoroughly in hot soapy water and dry completely before reusing them for your own recipes.

Squirt Bottles   Recycle liquid soap dispensers, dish washing liquid, and shampoo bottles for storing your homemade bath and massage oils, shampoos, and body splashes.

Tins   Tins make ideal storage facilities for dry recipes such as scrubs, masks, and bath crystal mixtures. They are generally airtight and keep out bugs, microscopic life, and light.

Zip-Seal Plastic Bags   If you have made a large quantity of a dry recipe, small or large plastic bags make ideal storage, and their contents can be kept fresh in a cool, dark place for several months.

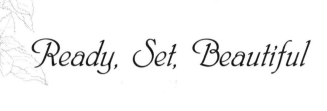

Ready, Set, Beautiful

You'll find many of the following items for applying beauty treatments around your home. What you don't own, you can easily purchase at pharmacies or supermarkets. Before applying any hair dyes, either wash your hair in warm water then towel off excess or apply to dry hair. Most conditioners are meant to be applied after shampooing. Read and follow the guidelines for application included in each recipe.

✍ Special Care for Sensitive Skin

Even basic natural ingredients can cause problems for some. Everyone's skin is unique. What might hurt one person might heal another. Just because the ingredient is natural doesn't mean that it can't cause a reaction. Lanolin; borax; essential flora, aromatic, and nut oils; and some other concentrated botanical extracts can cause a sore, puffy, oozing, red, or itchy reaction on the skin. It is essential to perform a skin patch test whenever a recipe calls for an ingredient you've never used before. If you have a known food allergy, assume you'll experience similar reactions when you apply that food to your skin in the form of a salve, cream, or moisturizer.

To perform a skin patch test, apply a small amount of the preparation on your thigh, upper arm, or breast, then cover with a Band-Aid or cotton gauze and leave it on overnight. Watch for itchiness, reddened rash, or irritation with puffiness or oozing secretions. If that happens, bathe the area with a weak solution of soda bicarbonate, then soothe with a lavish application of fresh aloe gel. Leave the skin to dry, then apply a salve of calendula or comfrey. Obviously, you'll want to avoid that recipe in the future.

❧ Tools

Complexion or Blush Brushes These are usually thick, rounded, soft-bristle brushes with short handles. They are used to apply facials, pastes, and masks. Be careful not to cover the sensitive skin around the lips and eyes.

Cotton Balls or Sterilized Cotton Squares These can be used to apply astringents, toners, nail oils, and eye refreshers. Cotton balls can be expensive, so I buy rolled-up cotton. I break off a small amount when a recipe calls for dabbing or compress application.

Loofah or Sea Sponge These sponges are ideal for applying exfoliating body scrubs and packs. Loofah is the dried skeleton of a gourd, which can be grown in your garden. You can also find loofahs in most health food and drug stores. The loofahs are too rough for delicate facial skin, so use dry sea sponges on the face.

Newspaper Some of the body packs and hair dyes are messy to make and apply, so cover your preparation surfaces completely with newspapers to prevent stains. You'll need to take the same special care when applying your recipes.

Cotton Diapers If the baby can spare a few, these make excellent compresses.

Tissues Use tissues to blot excess oil, perspiration, and lip makeup. Stick to unscented, 100 percent cotton tissues as dyes and fragrances can irritate delicate complexions.

Tinctures, Infusions, and Decoctions

ॐ Making Herbal Tinctures at Home

T inctures capture botanical properties of herbs, and you can store them for
years. They are easily absorbed through the deeper dermal layers. I make
tinctures for many of my bathing and massage recipes.

ॐ For Fresh Herbs

5 tablespoons fresh herb
1½ cups 100-proof vodka

Fill a dark-colored glass jar (16-oz. size is ideal) with the herb. Cover with the
vodka, right to the rim. Close tightly and label with the herb name, spirit base, and date
sealed. After three days, add more vodka, again to the rim of the jar, and reseal. Leave
tincture processing for 6 weeks, then strain through a fine mesh. Funnel herbal tincture

into 1-oz. glass bottles with glass dropper lids (for storage). Seal and label with contents and date.

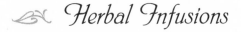 For Dried Herbs

5 tablespoons herb
1½ cups 100-proof vodka

Place the dried herb in a 16-oz. jar. Pour 1¼ cups vodka over the herb, then seal. Leave for one week, then top off with more vodka. Reseal and allow to process for 6–8 weeks. Strain herbs and pour into sterilized, small, dark-colored jars with glass dropper lids. Seal and label with contents and date. Store at room temperature, away from direct sunlight and damp. The tincture will remain potent for at least 3 years if resealed tightly after each use.

All of the following herbal preparations must be made in advance. The tinctures, macerated oils, and glycerins need to be made two months in advance of making the recipe that calls for it. The infusions and decocotions take only thirty minutes and can be used immediately. While the floral waters and vinegars are processing, they can add color and beauty to your home through the natural vibrations of the healing light rays they will give off. Remember to save all your herbal waste for the compost heap.

Herbal Infusions

I use herbal infusions for bathing, body mists, facial tonics, and hair rinses.

1 tablespoon dried herb leaves, seeds, and/or flowers (or 2 tablespoons fresh)
2 cups very hot water

Place the herb in a heat-resistant pitcher or bowl. Cover with hot water. Do not use boiling water, as the potency of the valuable living extracts will denature. The best way to heat water to the right temperature is with an electric kettle. I switch mine off just before it boils, then let it stand for 5 minutes. Cover herb matter for 15 minutes to steep. Strain through a fine mesh or cheesecloth, and funnel the infusion into a sterilized glass bottle. Either refrigerate (will keep for 5 days) or use immediately.

≈ *Bud Macerated Glycerin*

This simple preparation extracts valuable plant ingredients from the spring buds of trees, shrubs, and bushes that are preserved in a spirit base and glycerin. Like seeds, buds contain the highest concentration of active nutrients in the whole plant. Their growth tissues have powerful therapeutic and cosmetic values. I use this preparation for my antiaging recipes and bathing treats.

1 tablespoon fresh buds
1 cup vegetable glycerin
½ cup vodka

Carefully prune a few small branches of the plant, then snip about 20 perfectly formed buds. Place the buds into a blender with the vodka and glycerin. Blend on a low speed for 15 seconds, then on a high speed for another 15 seconds. Transfer the pureed mixture into a sterilized, dark-colored glass bottle. Fill to the brim, then seal tightly. Date, label, and shelve the bottle. The mixture will take 3 weeks to mature, but you'll need to shake the jar daily. Strain contents through a fine mesh or cheesecloth, then through a coffee filter paper, squeezing out as much liquid as possible. Pour the macerated glycerin into small, sterilized, 1-oz. dark-colored glass bottles with dropper lids, to the rim (to prevent oxidation). Seal and label with contents and date. If sealed and stored correctly, this preparation will keep for 2–3 years.

Buds that can be macerated using this technique:

Apple	Carrot	Lime
Beechnut	Cherry	Linden
Black, red, and white currant	Cobnut	Raspberry
	Horse chestnut	Rose
Black poplar	Lemon	Walnut

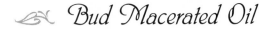 *Bud Macerated Oil*

There are two techniques to making this oil. I prefer to use the heat method, which is quicker and lasts longer.

8 tablespoons fresh herbs or flowers
1 cup olive oil
4 tablespoons dry white wine
Dark glass jar with dropper lid for storage

Put all the ingredients into a blender. Process for 30 seconds on a high speed, then 15 seconds on a low speed. Pour into a sterilized, shallow, dark-glass jar, to the rim. Seal tightly and place on a sunny windowsill for three weeks. Shake the jar daily. This action of shaking increases the rate at which the live botanical disperses into the oil. Pour mixture into a double boiler and gently heat through until all the wine has evaporated. Cool, then strain, first through a fine mesh, then a paper coffee filter. Funnel the remaining oil into 1-oz. sterilized bottles with dropper lids. Seal and label. These potent botanical extracts will remain fresh and active for up to 2 years.

Herbs that can be macerated using this technique:

Bay	Lavender	Rosemary
Carrot seed	Lemon balm	Sage
Chamomile	Linden flower	Saint-John's-wort
Comfrey	Linseed	Thyme
Dandelion	Marigold (calendula)	Yarrow
Fennel seed	Marjoram	
Geranium	Peppermint	

❧ Herbal Decoctions from Roots, Barks, and Berries

This technique, although used mainly to prepare herbal medicines, extracts the valuable botanicals from herb roots, barks, berries, and rhizomes through a process of boiling and simmering in water for over 30 minutes or until the liquid has reduced by a third. Most decoctions are prepared for immediate use, but they can be stored in the refrigerator for 2 days in a sealed bottle.

3 tablespoons herb

3 cups water

Combine ingredients and bring to a boil. Reduce the heat and simmer for 30 minutes or until the liquid has been reduced by one-third. Strain through a fine mesh and leave to cool before bottling. If you are not using it immediately, you can refrigerate an herbal decoction for 2 days.

Suggested herbs for decoctions:

Burdock root   Gingerroot

Comfrey root   Witch hazel bark

✍ Herbal Floral Waters

These floral waters (or hydrosols) are the wonderful, sensually aromatic additions to many of my beautiful-body recipes. During the short season when my garden herbs flower, I preserve their subtle fragrances and colors with this simple technique. I add them to refreshing body mists, moisturizers, and massage lotions. I store different floral waters in bottles of various sizes and line my study windowsill with a rainbow of healing colors.

2 cups fresh flowers

3 cups water

Place the flowers in a clear-glass bottle, then fill with water right up to the rim (to prevent oxidation). Seal and label with contents and date. Place in a sunny window for 4–6 weeks, shaking it from time to time to increase the rate at which the botanicals disperse into the water. Strain through a fine mesh, then pour into small (2- or 3-oz.) decorative glass bottles. Seal tightly, date, and label. Since these floral waters are less concentrated than pure essential oils, they can be used without diluting. If stored in airtight containers, they will remain potent for up to 2 or 3 months.

Floral Vinegar Splashes and Mists

On a hot summer day, I find it very refreshing to splash or mist my skin with these aromatic floral vinegars. Due to the natural process of fermentation, these floral vinegar recipes will remain potent for up to a year.

8 tablespoons fresh flower heads (chopped finely)
4 cups wine vinegar

Place the flowers into a sterilized glass jar, then completely cover with the wine vinegar (for red rose petals, use red wine vinegar). Allow to steep for 1 week, shaking the jar daily to increase the rate at which the botanical disperses into the vinegar. Strain through a fine mesh, then funnel into an attractive, sterilized, colored-glass bottle. Seal and label with contents and date.

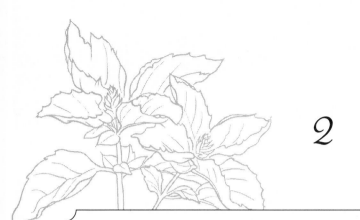

2

Recipes and Remedies

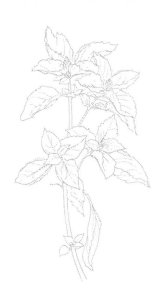

Facials

*A*ll skin types benefit from a special treat once in a while. Natural, living facials will leave your complexion glowing, and they're easy to make. Young complexions will benefit from a living facial once a month; more mature skins can use them up to twice a week. Facials speed the rate at which cells are regenerated. With regular facials, you'll have a younger-looking, more energized complexion.

Your skin accounts for approximately 15 percent of your body weight. One inch of skin contains approximately twenty million cells, seven hundred sweat glands, eighty heat and cold receptors, nine hundred pain receptors, twenty million sensory nerve cells, eighty hair follicles, and fifteen yards of blood vessels. Your skin is a living, breathing reflection of your diet and the way you care for it.

Exfoliating means removing the top layer of dead skin cells. Living facials are excellent and gentle exfoliants. These treatments also deep-clean pores. Facials should always be gentle, or your skin could end up looking like a mass of tiny, broken veins.

Before applying these living facials, undress your skin. Wash with warm water, then apply a diluted herbal cleanser. Massage 1 teaspoon of cold-pressed vegetable oil into your skin from your neck to your forehead. When applying your facial, be careful not to cover the sensitive skin around your lips and eyes. Rinse off each treatment with warm water. Then, if possible, air-dry outside or near an open window.

Annie's Herbal Steam and Facial

*T*his is a sensually aromatic recipe for a deep-cleansing herbal steam. It's good for oily and combination skin as it frees the sebaceous ducts and hair follicles of dirt and toxic impurities. The facial is penetrating and nourishing and is applied immediately after the herbal steam.

30 drops witch hazel (leaf) tincture

1 tablespoon each of the following herbs:

> Chamomile
>
> Lavender
>
> Lime
>
> Marigold flowers
>
> Rosemary
>
> Sage
>
> Thyme
>
> Walnut leaves

4 cups mineral water

3 tablespoons kaolin clay

10 drops calendula essential oil

3 drops lavender essential oil

Measure the tincture into a small bowl. Place the herbs into another bowl. Measure ⅔ cup of the mixed herbs and place into a saucepan. Add hot water, then cover and steep for 30 minutes. Strain a small amount of the warm infusion and mix 2 tablespoons of it with the kaolin clay to form a smooth paste. Set aside. Place the covered saucepan with the infused herbs on a table. You should be able to comfortably lean your head over it. Remove the cover, add the calendula and lavender essential oils and witch hazel tincture to the infusion and mix gently.

Lean over and place a large towel over your head, covering the saucepan and trapping the steam. After 5–10 minutes, remove the towel and lie down to cool off for 5 minutes. Using a spray bottle, mist your face with cold water, then splash your skin with a little of the remaining herbal infusion. Using a palette knife and your hands, apply the paste. Pile several layers over your chin, forehead, and nose.

Strain the infusion, discarding the herbs. Soak 3–5 cotton pads in the infusion, then place them over your pasted face and neck. Try not to flex your facial muscles by talking or twitching. Protect the area under your head with an old towel to catch any slides or drips. Remove cotton pads, rinse the mask with warm water. Pat dry.

Conclude this treatment with the following skin moisturizing lotion:

2 tablespoons freshly extracted (or unsweetened, preservative-free, bottled) grape juice

1 teaspoon cold-pressed almond or olive oil (for mature skins, use primrose oil)

Pour the juice and oil into a saucer. Dip 5–6 cotton balls into the mixture. Apply the lotion to your face. Allow the mixture to penetrate your skin. Leave it oil-dressed for at least 1 hour, and longer, if possible, before applying makeup. Better still, apply an hour before bed.

Chamomile-Oat Compress

This simple, effective recipe is especially beneficial for complexions that redden easily or become blotchy and irritated in cold weather. The oatmeal soothes skin and helps shrink capillaries. It also prevents tiny thread veins from forming beneath the skin's surface. Apply twice a week during the winter months, when your face is under constant attack. Adding 1 teaspoon of molasses to the warming paste before application gives it a gentle antiseptic property.

1 tablespoon finely ground oatmeal

½ cup mineral water

3 drops chamomile essential oil

1 cup cold mineral water (placed in a spray bottle)

1 bowl very hot water, 1 bowl of cold water (for application)

1 teaspoon molasses (optional)

Place the oatmeal in a small bowl and stir with ½ cup water. Allow the oatmeal to absorb the water and thicken into a paste. Add the chamomile essential oil, one drop at a time, stirring the mixture after adding each drop. When you are ready to apply the compress, you'll need 2 washcloths and the paste handy. Place the 2 bowls of water (one hot and one cold) on your application area. Cover your shoulders with an old towel and bind your hair off your face with a headband, if necessary. Mist your face and upper neck with the cold mineral water in a spray bottle. Dip a clean washcloth into the chamomile-oat paste, then dab it on your face. Keep dipping and dabbing until your face and neck are covered. Avoid the skin around your eyes and lips. Place another washcloth into the hot water to make a hot compress, and place it over your pasted face. Rest for 15 minutes. Remove washcloth and place it in the cold water. Repeat procedure. Rinse well, dry, and moisturize.

❧ Jane's Spring Orchard Facial

The humble apple and skin-soothing aloe are used together in this refreshing and skin-rejuvenating facial. It improves the complexion, counteracting premature photo-aging and other skin stressors. Try this wonderful facial twice a month. Its active, live enzymes consume surface bacteria and dislodge dead skin cells.

½ cup fresh aloe juice and gel (from 10 large leaves)

2 Granny Smith apples, cored and stemmed

2 egg whites

2 teaspoons cold-pressed almond oil

2 teaspoons cold-pressed wheat germ oil

10 drops marigold essential oil

3 tablespoons lemon juice (from 1 lemon)

Cut about 10 large leaves of aloe lengthwise. Using the blunt edge of a knife, scrape off the gel and juice and put it into a saucer. Mash the gel with a fork and set aside. Core and chop the apples and place in a blender with the egg whites, oils, and lemon juice. Blend at high speed for 30 seconds. Pour the mixture into a small bowl, then add the aloe and stir well. If the mixture is too dry, add a little more lemon juice.

To apply, bind your hair back off your face and forehead, if necessary. Spread the paste over your face and upper neck. Relax for 15 minutes. Rinse with warm water, then moisturize.

Exotic Fruit Facial

I make this wonderful treatment in the late spring and early summer months when seasonal fruit is plentiful and the herbs are young and flowering. This delicious facial firms skin, heals blemishes and soothes all skin types. Lime and yarrow buds can be collected from the open countryside, your garden, or purchased from organic herb suppliers.

½ ripe banana

1 peeled and stoned plum

1 large apple

3 small, pink apricots

25 drops lime bud macerated glycerin (to make bud macerated glycerin, see page 37)

25 drops yarrow macerated oil (to make bud macerated oil, see page 38)

1 tablespoon live-culture yogurt

2 teaspoons honey

1 tablespoon dried orrisroot (ground finely)

Core, seed, stone, and chop the fruits and place in the blender. Add the glycerin, oil, yogurt, honey, and orrisroot. Blend on a high speed for 30 seconds. If the mixture is too runny, add more orrisroot and mix to a paste consistency. Apply, using your hands or an old pastry or makeup brush. Generously cover your forehead, chin, nose, and neck. Leave on for 30 minutes. Rinse thoroughly with warm water and pat dry. Apply a skin-nourishing moisturizer.

Pore-Tight Mask

I created this simple mask for my brother, who suffered from acne most of his teenage life. He was a little reluctant to try a facial, something he considered decidedly feminine, but finally decided to try it (behind locked doors of course). Within days, he noticed a difference. With a few changes in his diet, he regained his childlike, clear complexion. This facial is especially beneficial for oily and combination skin types. Use it twice a week. Increase the benefits of this treatment by eliminating all fried foods, saturated fats, refined flours, and processed foods from your diet. Remember, your skin is a reflection of the food you eat.

1 egg white

1 tablespoon distilled witch hazel solution

1 tablespoon fuller's earth

Lightly beat the egg white in a small bowl, then set aside. In a second bowl, combine the witch hazel and fuller's earth and mix into a smooth paste. Fold into the beaten egg white and beat vigorously. To apply, bind your hair off your forehead and face. Apply the paste with your hands or an old makeup brush. Cover your whole face, leaving large bare-skin circles around your lips and eyes. Leave on for 30 minutes. Rinse with warm water, pat dry, and apply a light, skin-nourishing moisturizer.

Rosy Facial

One of my grandmother's secrets to her clear, soft complexion was the weekly application of this sweet-smelling, feminine facial. Its slightly gritty texture gently buffs the skin's surface, dislodging dead skin cells, while the honey and oatmeal cleanse and heal. The rose water refreshes and tones. Before applying this facial, my grandmother always misted her face and neck with a refreshing infusion of spearmint and chamomile flowers, which she picked fresh from her garden. Try the Chamomile-Ginseng Skin Mist on page 62.

FACIAL

1 teaspoon honey

3 teaspoons granulated sugar

2 tablespoons pure rose water

2 tablespoons medium-ground oatmeal

Measure and mix the honey, sugar, rose water, and oatmeal in a bowl. Vigorously beat into a gritty paste. Before you apply, mist your face and neck with the chilled infusion. Allow it to air-dry. Then, using your hands, gently smooth the facial over your skin, leaving large, bare circles around your eyes and lips. Gently massage with your fingertips for about 5 minutes. Rinse with warm water, pat dry, then moisturize.

❧ Queenie's Honey-Barley Mask

This simple, skin-nourishing recipe refines and moisturizes while tightening slack facial tissues. Barley is an excellent skin food, whether ingested in the form of a hot tea or combined with fresh orange or lemon juice as a refreshing and cool beverage. This recipe uses barley flour as a gentle exfoliant. The addition of gelatin lets you peel off the mask. Along with it goes embedded debris and dead skin cells.

½ cup pear juice

1 tablespoon unflavored gelatin

⅓ cup organic barley flour

2 tablespoons clear honey

1 egg white

Mix the juice and gelatin powder together in the top of a double boiler, or mix the juice and gelatin powder in a bowl and microwave for 45 seconds on high. Refrigerate for 20 minutes. Meanwhile, in a separate bowl, mix the barley flour and honey into a stiff paste. Beat the egg white gently and add to the barley-honey mixture.

To apply, use your hands to smooth the barley paste over your face and neck. Next, layer on the gelatin mixture. Relax for 30 minutes. Warm your hands in hot water and press them to your face to soften the hardened mask. Peel the mask off. Rinse with warm water, pat dry. Apply a light skin-nourishing moisturizer.

Moisturizing Mask

The nutrients in this skin-food mask are rapidly absorbed and go directly where they are needed. It contains natural lecithin from egg yolks that locks moisture to the skin. Yogurt contains lactic acid, another excellent moisture-fixing ingredient. When used regularly, this mask can fade freckles and age spots.

2 tablespoons plain, live-culture yogurt

1 fresh egg yolk

½ teaspoon clear blossom honey

1 teaspoon mayonnaise

Measure the ingredients into a small bowl and mix into a smooth paste. Bind your hair off your face with a towel. Using your hands, spread the mask over your skin, leaving bare-skin circles around your eyes and mouth. Relax for 30 minutes. Rinse off with warm water. Pat dry. Leave the skin undressed overnight.

Fruit Facial and Skin Wash

When applied to the skin, active antioxidants in fruits and vegetables have many revitalizing, toning, soothing, and stimulating effects. The alpha-hydroxy acids (AHAs) found in pineapple and melon work their special magic by correcting the skin's pH and allowing it to slough off dead skin cells. The kaolin is deeply penetrating and, in combination with the other ingredients, leaves the skin toned, refreshed, and silky soft.

4 oz. fresh pineapple

4 oz. ripe watermelon (with seeds)

2 oz. pear (with skin)

1 teaspoon comfrey root (powdered)

2 tablespoons kaolin powder

Gently wash the fruit. Chop into small chunks and place in a blender. Process on a high speed for 30 seconds, then add the comfrey root and kaolin. Blend for another 15 seconds on a low speed. If the mixture is too stiff, add 1 teaspoon of honey. If it's too runny, add a little more kaolin. Make the chamomile infusion (see page 36), allowing it to steep for 15 minutes.

To apply, use your hands to smooth the mask on your skin. Pile several layers over your chin, forehead, nose, and upper neck. Relax for 30 minutes, rinse with warm water, and pat dry.

SKIN WASH

½ cup goat's milk

3 drops marigold essential oil

½ cup chamomile infusion (warm)

Whisk ingredients together in a bowl. After thoroughly rinsing the facial and drying your skin, add the milk and essential oil to the strained, warm chamomile infusion and splash your face, leaving it to dry on your skin overnight.

❧ Trudi's Combination Skin Mask

This simple mask is one of my favorites. Apples help to firm the skin, while lemons have an age-old reputation for boosting the micro-circulation of the skin. Both are rich in antioxidants, making them excellent remedies for wrinkles. The live enzymatic action of the fresh pulp tightens the pores, while gently exfoliating. The oatmeal and yogurt soothe and stimulate.

> 1 small cored and grated apple (with skin)
> 2 teaspoons lemon juice
> 2 tablespoons finely ground oatmeal
> 1 tablespoon plain yogurt

Place the grated apple and lemon juice into a small bowl, mix the yogurt in with a fork, then sprinkle the oatmeal over the wet mixture. Stir to form a smooth paste.

Use your hands to spread the paste over your face and upper neck. Relax for 20 minutes, then rinse with warm water. Pat dry with a warm towel, then moisturize.

❧ Minty-Oats and Aloe Skin Refresher

Peppermint peps up the skin's tone and has a stimulating and firming effect. Aloe is slightly astringent but very soothing to the skin's surface. This easy-to-make facial acts as a natural humectant and light exfoliant, healing minor irritations.

> 1 teaspoon freshly chopped peppermint leaves (or ½ teaspoon dried peppermint leaves)
> 4 tablespoons finely ground oatmeal

Beautiful Face, Beautiful Body

4 tablespoons very hot (not boiling) water

2 teaspoons aloe juice/gel

Gently wash the peppermint leaves. If you are using dried leaves, place them in a small bowl and barely cover them with hot water. Steep for 5 minutes and drain. Chop the fresh or hydrated leaves finely. Sprinkle the oatmeal over the peppermint leaves and add the hot water. Set aside for 5 minutes. Add the aloe, then mix well.

Use your hands or an old makeup brush to smooth the paste over your face, leaving bare-skin circles around your eyes and mouth. Relax for 30 minutes. Try not to flex your facial muscles by talking or twitching. Rinse with warm water and pat dry. Apply a light moisturizer.

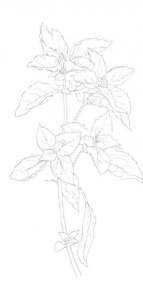

Mists and Splashes

*T*here is nothing more important for healthy, young-looking skin than water. Healthy skin is hydrated skin. Drinking plenty of water (at least two liters every day) is essential to maintaining skin firmness and tone. That's hydrating from the inside out. Treat your skin from the outside in with everything from moisturizing facials and cleansers to the mists and splashes from the pages that follow.

There's nothing quite as refreshing on a hot summer day as a facial mist, but don't wait for the hot summer sun to indulge yourself with these recipes. I always begin my facial routine with a thorough cleansing followed by a drenching mist of an herbal infusion. I use skin soothing mists before applying abrasive scrubs and packs, and mildly astringent splashes afterward. I can't get enough of them!

Chamomile-Ginseng Skin Mist

2 tablespoons fresh chamomile flowers (or 3 tea bags)

3 ginseng root tea bags

1 cup very hot (but not boiling) water

Place the fresh chamomile flowers (or tea bags) and the ginseng tea bags into a small pint-sized pitcher. Cover with the water and steep for 30 minutes. Once cool, strain through a fine mesh (or squeeze out the bags) and pour into a spritzer bottle. Refrigerate for 10 minutes. Use to moisten skin before your favorite facial.

Comfrey-Marigold Skin Wash

1 tablespoon chopped comfrey root

1 tablespoon fresh marigold flowers

1 tablespoon fresh chamomile flowers

2 cups very hot water

Steep herbs in hot water for 30 minutes. Strain and cool. Wash your face with this fragrant infusion and air-dry. Leftovers can be stored in the refrigerator for 2 days. Warm through before each use.

Rose Hip Mist

1 teaspoon rose hip berries

1 teaspoon chamomile flowers

1 cup very hot (not boiling) water

Steep rose hips and chamomile flowers in hot water for 20 minutes. Strain and cool. Pour into a spray bottle and mist over your face and upper neck each night before applying moisturizer.

Lavender Fizz

30 drops lavender
½ cup sparkling water

Combine oil and water. Leave closed in a bottle kept in the dark for 2 days. Strain through coffee filter paper, blotting out oil and leaving its aromatic properties in the water. Splash over skin and allow to dry before applying geranium moisturizer. It's so refreshing!

Rose Hip–Comfrey Mist

4 tablespoons chamomile infusion
4 tablespoons rose hip infusion
4 tablespoons comfrey root infusion

Follow instructions for making floral infusions (page 36) and let each steep, covered, for 1 hour. Strain. Pour together into a spray bottle and refrigerate for 10 minutes. Mist your face and neck with this refreshing, skin-nourishing infusion before cleansing.

Burdock Facial Mist

1 cup burdock root decoction
4 tablespoons fresh carrot juice

Place 1 heaped tablespoon of chopped burdock root in 3 cups of water in a saucepan. Bring to a boil, then simmer for 15 minutes (until water has reduced by one-third). Strain and either eat the delicious vegetable or discard it. Pour 1 cup of the decoction into a spray bottle along with the fresh carrot juice. Refrigerate for 15 minutes. Spray on your skin after cleansing.

Flower Water Mist

3 tablespoons violet flower water

3 tablespoons lavender flower water

3 tablespoons orange flower water

Make the flower waters by placing 1 cup of each flower (separately) in 3 cups of water. Bruise the flowers by pressing them with the back of a wooden spoon. Bottle and seal the three flower waters and leave on a sunny windowsill for 2 weeks, shaking daily to increase the process of botanicals dispersing into the water. Strain, discarding the flowers, then combine the waters in a spray bottle. Mist your face and neck.

Rose Hip–Chamomile Mist

4 tablespoons rose hip infusion

4 tablespoons chamomile infusion

4 tablespoons calendula infusion

Take one tea bag of each herb and immerse each in its own cup of very hot water. Cover and steep for 30 minutes. Squeeze out the bags and save for composting. Funnel an equal measure of each infusion into a spray bottle. Leave to chill in the refrigerator for 5 minutes. Mist your upper body thoroughly.

Beautiful Face, Beautiful Body

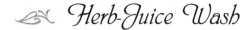
Herb-Juice Wash

4 tablespoons calendula flower infusion

4 tablespoons lavender flower infusion

1 teaspoon fresh watercress juice

Make the flower infusions as above. Steep, covered, for 30 minutes. Strain through a fine mesh. Pour into a bowl, then add the watercress juice. Beat gently with a whisk. To apply, place a clean washcloth into the infusion, then use the wet cloth to wash your skin.

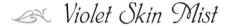
Comfrey-Elderflower Skin Mist

4 tablespoons comfrey leaf and root decoction

4 tablespoons elderflower infusion

4 tablespoons red grape juice

Follow the instructions for making a flower infusion (page 36) and root decoction (page 39) then cover and allow to steep for 2 hours. Strain, then mix with the fresh grape juice. Funnel into a spray bottle and mist upper body generously.

Violet Skin Mist

3 teaspoons violet flower water

1 tablespoon distilled witch hazel solution

6–8 drops benzoin tincture (found in drug stores)

Funnel the violet flower water and witch hazel solution into a spray bottle, then add the benzoin tincture. Shake well. Refrigerate for 5 minutes. Mist over cleansed skin and air-dry.

✍ *Aromatic Vinegar Wash*

1 tablespoon rose petals

1 teaspoon lavender flowers

1 teaspoon jasmine flowers

4 cups white wine vinegar

1 cup rose water

Place the flowers in a sterilized glass bottle, then use a funnel to pour the vinegar over the flowers. Seal and steep for 3 days, shaking the contents from time to time. Then mix the contents of the bottle with the rose water, rebottle, and place in a sunny window. After 4 days, strain contents through a fine mesh, then rebottle. Pour 1 tablespoon of the aromatic vinegar wash into a bowl and add 1 cup of warm water. Splash on all over, then pat dry.

✍ *Dandelion Flower Mist*

1 tablespoon fresh dandelion petals

1 tablespoon fresh chamomile flowers

1 tablespoon fresh marigold petals

2 cups very hot water

Immerse flowers in the water. Cover and steep for 1 hour. Strain, then funnel into a spray bottle and refrigerate for 15 minutes.

Orange Flower Refresher

3 tablespoons orange flower water

1 tablespoon fresh orange juice

2 drops calendula essential oil

1 cup water

Gently whisk the ingredients in a bowl then funnel into a spray bottle and refrigerate for 5 minutes.

Lavender Vinegar Splash

½ cup fresh lavender flowers

1 cup white wine vinegar

1 cup mineral water

Place lavender flowers into a glass jar, then funnel in the vinegar. Seal and label. Leave for 1 week, shaking the jar from time to time. Strain 1 tablespoon into a bowl and mix with 1 cup water. Splash floral vinegar over exfoliated skin, then air-dry.

Ginseng Mist

4 tablespoons ginseng root infusion

4 tablespoons distilled witch hazel solution

1 cup warm mineral water

Put 4 ginseng tea bags into a 2 cups of very hot water. Cover and steep for 30 minutes, then strain. Funnel the measured amount of the infusion with the distilled witch hazel and 1 cup of mineral water into a spritzer bottle.

✑ Orange-Lavender Mist

2 tablespoons freshly squeezed orange juice

4 tablespoons distilled rose water

2 drops lavender

2 drops bergamot

½ cup warm water

Strain orange juice, then funnel into a spray bottle with the other ingredients. Shake vigorously before each use so that oils and juice are thoroughly mixed.

✑ Calendula Skin Spray

4 tablespoons chamomile infusion

4 tablespoons calendula infusion

4 tablespoons comfrey infusion

Make an infusion of the combined herbs following the instructions on page 36. Cover and steep for 1 hour, then strain. Funnel into a spray bottle.

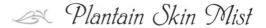# Plantain Skin Mist

1 tablespoon fennel seeds and leaves

1 tablespoon plantain leaves and flowers

1 tablespoon cornflowers

Follow the instructions for making herbal infusions on page 36. Allow infusion to steep, covered, for 1 hour. Strain through a fine mesh. Funnel into a spray bottle, then gently mist your face and eyes.

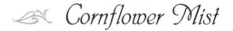# Cornflower Mist

4 tablespoons cornflower infusion (see instructions page 36)

½ cup sparkling mineral water

Combine and pour into spray bottle. Mist generously to refresh and nourish your eyes.

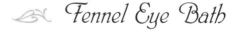# Fennel Eye Bath

3 tablespoons fennel seed infusion

Make the fennel seed infusion by placing 2 teaspoons of dried seed in 1 cup of very hot mineral water. Cover and steep for 30 minutes. Strain, then chill in the refrigerator for 10 minutes. Soak cotton balls or sterilized gauze into the fennel infusion and dab on any creases around the mouth, eyes, nose, and chin. Leave to air-dry.

Herb Milk Mist

½ cup buttermilk

1 tablespoon marshmallow root (powdered)

Slowly heat the buttermilk and marshmallow root in a saucepan. Simmer for 15 minutes. Strain and cool. Splash over your face before applying your favorite facial treatment.

Fruit Juice Mist

¼ cup fresh carrot juice

¼ cup fresh apricot juice

1 tablespoon aloe juice

Extract the carrot and apricot juices, then whip in the aloe juice. Funnel into a spray bottle and refrigerate. Mist your face and upper neck.

Comfrey-Apricot Mist

½ cup chamomile flower infusion (see instructions on page 36)

2 tablespoons comfrey root decoction (see instructions on page 39)

4 tablespoons fresh apricot juice

First make the facial mist. Combine the chamomile infusion in a bowl with the comfrey root decoction and apricot juice. Place in the refrigerator for 10 minutes, then funnel into a spray bottle and lavishly mist your face and neck.

Marigold Flower Mist

4 tablespoons dandelion flower infusion

4 tablespoons marigold flower infusion

2 tablespoons plantain leaf infusion

Make the herbal infusions following the instructions on page 36. Strain through a fine mesh, then funnel into a spray bottle. Refrigerate for 5 minutes before use.

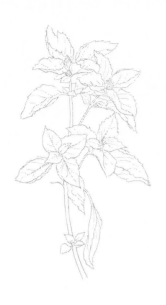

Moisturizers

Your skin has the natural ability to keep itself moist. It combines natural secretions (sebum) with water that it extracts from the immediate environment. Sebum is secreted through your pores by the billions of glands beneath your skin's surface. It is naturally acidic and has antibacterial properties that protect the skin's surface from germs.

Hormonal variations affect sebum production and distribution, which is one reason why skin types vary so much. Normal skin types are basically balanced all over, with no areas of excessive secretions. Dry skin types have an inadequate oil secretion. Combination skin types usually have an overproduction of oil secretion around the nose, mouth, chin, and forehead. Oily skin types have an overproduction and distribution of oil secretions all over the face. The moisture level of your skin is affected by variables including weather conditions, diet, water consumption, humidity, and sun exposure. All these factors contribute to skin hydration or dehydration, which can cause premature aging.

Natural, living moisturizers and skin protectors top off the skin's moisture levels by forming a protective film over the surface, preventing valuable water loss. There are two main types of moisturizers: water-in-oil and oil-in-water. Water-in-oil moisturizers are richly nourishing creams and lotions that suit dry, sensitive skin types. More mature skin also benefits from these formulas. Deeply enriching moisturizers are especially useful during cold-weather months, when the skin is prone to cracking, chapping, and flaking. Oil-in-water formulas are easily absorbed and much lighter. They're suitable for combination, oily, and normal skin types.

The best time to apply a moisturizer is after showering or cleansing your face. If your skin has a tendency to dehydrate quickly, apply one of these herbal or skin-nourishing moisturizers to damp skin. The best type of nighttime moisturizer is one that contains living, skin-rejuvenating ingredients, with soothing botanical extracts that can easily penetrate the deeper skin layers while you sleep. With sufficient internal hydration and surface protection, your skin will maintain its natural moisture levels and soft texture.

Linda's Elderflower Moisturizer

Generations of women have distilled and infused their own elderflowers and used the solution on their skin as a daily cleanser. Elderflower is stimulating and mildly astringent. Many believe it whitens the skin, fading freckles and age spots. This recipe is an especially refreshing after-bath splash. It encapsulates moisture droplets, which are then absorbed by the skin. Used regularly, this sweet-scented moisturizer will give you a wonderfully soft complexion.

1 ½ cups elderflower infusion (to make an infusion, see instructions on page 36)
1 tablespoon beeswax pearls
5 tablespoons cocoa butter
½ cup sweet almond oil
7 drops lavender essential oil

Make the infusion, steep, strain in a bowl, and set aside to cool. Meanwhile, place the beeswax, cocoa butter, and almond oil into a double boiler and heat until melted. Once cooled, blend the oily mixture, then add to the elderflower infusion and beat vigorously. Add the lavender essential oil, one drop at a time, stirring after each drop is added. After showering or bathing, splash the elderflower moisturizer over your still-moist skin. Massage, using sweeping, upward movements. Store any excess in a shallow jar. Discard after 4 weeks.

Butter-Chamomile Cream

Chamomile is an age-old skin remedy. It soothes, heals, combats inflammation, and stimulates cell regeneration. It is rich in a fatty substance called azulene, which possesses extraordinary antibacterial, anti-inflammatory, and healing powers. Cocoa butter is an excellent skin barrier. Together, these ingredients bind, cleanse, and protect the skin from many environmental pollutants. Use an herbal infusion, such as the Comfrey Skin Wash (page 62) as a refreshing cleanser before applying the cream.

    1 tablespoon beeswax pearls
    3 tablespoons cocoa butter
    4 tablespoons cold-pressed avocado oil
    4 tablespoons cold-pressed jojoba bean oil
    1 tablespoon clear honey
    12 drops chamomile *(Matricaria recutita)* essential oil

Place the wax and oils into the top of a double boiler until melted. Remove from the heat and set aside until cool. Then stir in the honey and beat gently. Add the chamomile essential oil, one drop at a time, stirring the mixture as each drop is added. Sparingly massage cream into skin daily.

✍ Josephine's Linseed Moisturizer

Before going to bed, lavishly apply this richly aromatic and skin-nourishing moisturizer. It penetrates the deeper dermal layers as you sleep. Linseeds are an excellent source of natural mucilage, a gel-like paste that soothes the skin's surface. The neroli essential oil gives this moisturizer a sensual aroma. Before applying, use an herbal mist, such as the Rose Hip Mist (page 62).

2 tablespoons cracked linseeds

1 cup very hot water

1 tablespoon vegetable glycerin

1 tablespoon rose water

3 drops neroli (orange flower) essential oil

Crack the linseeds in a coffee grinder or food processor for a few seconds. Place them in a bowl and pour in the hot water. Cover and allow to steep for 15 minutes. Stir, then strain. Discard the hulls and place the gel-like paste into a small bowl. Beat in the glycerin and rose water. Last, add the neroli essential oil, one drop at a time, stirring the mixture after each drop is added. Transfer into a sterilized glass bottle, seal, and label with contents and date.

Natural sunscreens are the best antiwrinkle products. Using a sunblock protects the skin from harmful free radicals, encouraging cell repair and regeneration. Block out UVA (long wavelength radiation), which is responsible for burning the deeper skin layers during the tanning process, and UVB (short wavelength radiation), responsible for surface sunburn, by wearing an SPF (sun protecting filter) daily, especially during the summer months. You should use sunscreen on your skin all year through, as ultraviolet rays can penetrate haze and shady spots, bounce off snow and water, and can even penetrate two feet of water.

Sensitive Complexion Sunscreen

This natural, living sunblock has particles that reflect back the sun's harmful UVA (long wavelength radiation) and UVB (short wavelength radiation). Apply it to your skin 20 minutes before sun exposure, as it takes that long for the protective ingredients to penetrate the deeper skin layers. This sunscreen is water-resistant and perfect for swimming. It can be used for all skin types, even babies' delicate skin.

> 2 tablespoon cold-pressed castor oil
> 4 tablespoons zinc oxide
> 1 tablespoon arrowroot powder

In a small bowl, mix the castor oil and zinc oxide into a smooth paste. Sprinkle the arrowroot over the oil paste and mix again. Transfer into a sterilized, small, shallow glass jar and seal tightly. This recipe is enough for 5 applications, but you can double or triple the ingredients for a weeklong beach vacation. Any skin not dressed in clothing should be dressed in this sunscreen, including toes, the tops of ears, lips, and noses.

Sun Worshipper Sunscreen

For those who just refuse to give up lounging in the burning sunshine (many of you tan easily), this simple, living sunscreen can be used all over the body. It contains natural tannins and oils that shield the skin from one-third of the sun's harmful rays. Sensitive, fair complexions, redheads, and children should use a stronger sunblock, such as the Sensitive Complexion Sunscreen (see above).

¼ cup Darjeeling infusion (black tea)

½ cup cold-pressed sesame oil

2 tablespoons cold-pressed jojoba bean oil

1 tablespoon cold-pressed avocado oil

Make the Darjeeling infusion by placing 5 tea bags into 3 cups of very hot (not boiling) water. Leave covered to steep for 30–60 minutes. Strain by squeezing out bags (save for composting) and pour liquid into a sterilized glass bottle. Measure ¼ cup of the infusion and pour into a bowl (discard the remaining tea). Add the oils and whip vigorously. Pour your sunscreen into a sterilized squirt bottle and store at room temperature. Shake well before each use. Massage lavishly on your exposed skin before and after swimming.

∂ *Agnes's Indian Sun Oil*

Full of exotic aromas, this wonderful, enriching oil goes on easily and will give you all-day protection. It's suitable for all skin types. Note that this is not a sunblock, so if you have a fair complexion and your skin burns easily, try the Sensitive Complexion Sunscreen on page 78.

1 tablespoon tahini

2 tablespoons coconut oil

1 teaspoon shea butter

1 tablespoon lanolin

½ cup strong Darjeeling infusion (black tea)

5 drops ylang ylang essential oil

Place the tahini, coconut oil, shea butter, and lanolin into the top of a double boiler and heat until melted. Stir occasionally. Meanwhile, make the Darjeeling infusion by immersing 5 tea bags into 2 cups of very hot water. Cover and steep for 30 minutes.

Squeeze out the bags and measure ½ cup of the tea (discard the remainder). Pour infusion into a sterilized, shallow glass jar, then add the cooled, melted mixture. Add the ylang ylang oil and stir. Seal and shake vigorously. Store at room temperature, discarding any left over after 6 weeks. At least 20 minutes before going outdoors, cover any skin that will be exposed. Lightly massage, using small, circular sweeping motions from your toes on up. Reapply after bathing or working up a sweat. Shake contents well before each use.

ᴈ Vicky's Geranium Moisturizer

This emollient moisturizer makes a delicious, sweet-smelling, nighttime treatment or a rich daily lotion for the whole body. Easily absorbed, it suits even the most sensitive skin types.

¼ cup cold-pressed avocado oil

2 tablespoons cold-pressed wheat germ oil

4 tablespoons cold-pressed jojoba bean oil

2 teaspoons shea butter

1 teaspoon beeswax pearls

2 tablespoons rose water

1 teaspoon borax powder

10 drops geranium essential oil

Combine the avocado, wheat germ, and jojoba oils in the top of a double boiler. Warm through, then add the shea butter and beeswax. Continue to stir the mixture until melted. Remove from the heat to cool. In a separate bowl, stir the rose water and borax until the borax dissolves. When the oily mixture has cooled, add to the rose water solution. Beat mixture vigorously. Add the geranium essential oil one drop at a time, stirring the mixture after each drop is added. Transfer into small, sterilized, shallow jars. Drench skin with an herbal splash, such as the Lavender Fizz (page 63) before applying geranium moisturizer.

✍ Calendula and Aloe Eye Balm

Botanical extracts, natural plant oils, and honey come together to moisturize the fragile tissues around the eyes. This balm soothes and will, to some extent, eliminate formation of wrinkles and laughter lines.

1 teaspoon cocoa butter
2 teaspoons cold-pressed wheat germ oil
1 teaspoon aloe gel
1 teaspoon lavender blossom honey
5 drops calendula essential oil

Place the cocoa butter and wheat germ oil in the top half of a double boiler. Heat until the cocoa butter has melted. Remove from heat and set aside until cool. Add the aloe gel and honey and beat vigorously. Add the calendula essential oil last, stirring the mixture as each drop is added. Use your fingertips to gently dab the balm to the delicate skin under and around your eyes, from the inner corners to the outer edges. Repeat massage on the upper lids. Use daily.

✍ Skin Food Moisturizer

This recipe smells good enough to eat (don't!) and feels so rich and luxurious that you just know that your skin is being nourished from the outside in. The oats and barley are exfoliating and skin-softening, while the oils penetrate and absorb into the deep (often malnourished) skin layers.

1 teaspoon shea butter

2 teaspoons cold-pressed wheat germ oil

½ teaspoon evening primrose oil

1 teaspoon cocoa butter

1 teaspoon beeswax pearls

½ cup barley and oat tea

1 teaspoon fresh aloe gel

Heat the first 5 ingredients in the top of a double boiler until melted, stirring occasionally. Make the barley and oat tea by placing 2 tablespoons of barley and oats into a saucepan half filled with cold water. Bring to a boil, then simmer for 10 minutes. Stir the mixture to keep it from sticking to the bottom of the pan. Remove from the heat, and strain the creamy, white liquid into a small glass bowl. Refrigerate. Combine the oil mixture with the cooled tea. Beat vigorously with a hand whisk, add aloe gel, and beat again. Any leftovers can be stored in a squeeze bottle. Using your fingertips, dab a little Skin Food Moisturizer onto your face and massage gently into your skin just before going to bed.

✥ Susy's Body Butter

Here's another concentrated body lotion that smells as good as it feels. It is packed with natural seed and nut butters that moisturize, condition, and gently exfoliate. It will leave your skin feeling as smooth as silk.

1 teaspoon coconut oil

2 teaspoons cold-pressed sesame seed oil

1 teaspoon shea butter

1 tablespoon cocoa butter

2 tablespoons cold-pressed avocado oil

1 teaspoon beeswax pearls

2 drops sandalwood essential oil

2 drops rosemary essential oil

Heat the first 6 ingredients in the top half of a double boiler until melted. Remove from the heat and beat vigorously with a hand whisk, then set aside to cool. Add the sandalwood and rosemary essential oils, one drop at a time, stirring the mixture after each drop is added. After bathing or showering, massage the body butter lotion over your still-moist skin. Use sweeping, circular motions, and cover the skin from your neck to your feet (and all the curves and creases in between).

❧ Rose Moisturizing Skin Splash

Simple and effective, this delightfully scented moisturizer glides on moistened skin, leaving it soft and supple. It makes an ideal skin splash for hot, humid, summer days. This moisturizer also offers a delicious psychological lift and tones the capillaries just beneath the skin's surface.

4 tablespoons vegetable glycerin

1 teaspoon cold-pressed wheat germ oil

8 tablespoons rose water

1 teaspoon fresh aloe gel

2 drops rose essential oil

2 drops myrtle essential oil

2 drops rockwood essential oil

Lightly whisk the glycerin, wheat germ oil, and rose water. Mix in the aloe and essential oils, one drop at a time, stirring after each drop. After showering, apply this splash all over in the warm, steamy air. Massage gently, using circular, sweeping motions all over your body and face. Towel off excess.

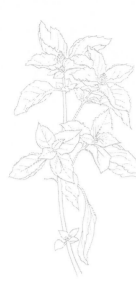

Cleansers and Tonics

*W*ashing with traditional soaps temporarily disrupts natural oil balance and production and can lead to overdryness or irritated blemish eruptions. Soap combines with calcium and magnesium deposits in hard water and leaves a nasty scum around the wash basin. Guess what? That same residue dries on your delicate skin. Once upon a time, commercial soap was considered the only option for people with oily and combination skin types due to its quick-drying effect. Strong, medicated soaps, which contain many harsh detergents, can worsen skin irritation. Their aggressive antiseptic agents and actions can cause chapping, flaking, and roughness. Many simply aren't very good at combating the more serious skin conditions such as persistent acne, dry erupted blemishes, and blackheads.

Many traditional commercial soaps are made from beef tallow or vegetable fats such as palm kernel and coconut oil, which encourage a thick lather. These soaps are highly alkaline, which in itself encourages complexion problems. The delicate pH of facial skin is between 4.5 and 6.5 pH, but these soaps raise it to 8.5 to 9.5 pH, sometimes even higher. The pH (potential hydrogen) refers to the skin's degree of acidity or alkalinity. The pH scale goes from 0 to 14, with a neutral point being 7 pH. Anything lower than 7 is regarded as acidic (the lower the pH, the greater the degree of acidity). Any reading above 7 is regarded as alkaline (the higher the pH, the greater the degree of alkalinity).

All of the following natural, living cleansers and beautifying tonics contain milder, more refreshing ingredients than commercial soaps. They are all simple to make. The difference you'll notice in your skin's tone and texture after using homemade soaps even for a few days will encourage you to create more inexpensive beauty cleansing preparations for yourself and your family. With the recipes in this chapter, you will be able to fill your bathroom cabinets with impressive, inexpensive beauty cleansing preparations for you and your family. By using a natural tonic or cleanser to keep your skin at its proper pH, you will prevent bacterial penetration (a result of too-acidic skin) and flaking and scaling due to moisture loss (a result of overly alkaline skin).

Millie's Spotty Skin Tonic

This refreshing skin tonic is made with a combination of stimulating ingredients. Lemon juice contains 7 percent citric and acts on the skin pores, making them appear smaller by puffing up the skin around them. Peppermint peps the skin, and the tea tree oil is gently antiseptic.

    4 tablespoons distilled witch hazel solution

    2 teaspoons lemon juice (1 small lemon)

    2 drops tea tree esential oil

    1 drop peppermint essential oil

Mix all the ingredients together by whipping with a hand whisk. Place in the refrigerator for 5 minutes before applying. Use in one application.

Skin Exfoliant Wash Balls

These wonderful skin helpers are so simple to make that they will become an indispensable part of your daily regimen. They naturally exfoliate the skin's surface while moisturizing and soothing minor skin irritations. I make these wonderful little unscented bath balls for my children. As a treat for myself, I add a few drops of chamomile, lavender, and ylang ylang essential oils to the dry mixture before securing it in the panty hose.

    3½ cups finely ground oat bran

    1 pair clean panty hose without holes (makes 6 balls)

Place the oat bran in a large bowl. Cut the legs off a pair of panty hose, discarding the panty. Fill the foot of one leg with about 4 tablespoons of oat bran. Leave the oat bran loosely packed, then secure with a knot. Remember to knot the cut end of the panty hose before filling with more of the oat mixture. Repeat this procedure twice, then fill the other leg the same way. You'll have six small oat bags.

Some variations: Add one of the following ingredients to each ball before securing with a knot.

1. 1 teaspoon of goat's milk (packed with skin-nourishing lactic acids).
2. 1 teaspoon of fresh lavender flowers (uplifting and slightly antiseptic).
3. 1 teaspoon fresh chamomile flowers (stimulating and cell-regenerating).

And that's it. Drop one ball in the running bathwater. Immerse yourself, and begin washing your skin with the delicate oat milk and soothing botanicals. You can use them while showering or place one in a basin of hot water, leave it to soak for 10 minutes, then splash wash your skin with the soothing milk.

Charlie's Medicated Rose Hip and Lavender Bar

This is an inexpensive, mildly antiseptic cleansing bar, ideal for acne-prone skin types and to soothe minor skin irritations. Attention nursing mothers: This cleansing bar heals nipples that are sore or cracked from mastitis or breast-feeding. It does not produce a frothy lather, but it is an excellent and refreshing purifier.

¼ cup sage leaf infusion
2 tablespoons lavender flower infusion

1 cup grated green Marseille olive oil soap

1 teaspoon vegetable oil (to grease the molds)

1 tablespoon rose hip seed oil *(Rosa rubiginosa)*

5 drops peppermint essential oil

5 drops tea tree essential oil

Follow the instructions for making sage and lavender infusions (page 36), cover, and steep separately overnight. Melt the grated soap in the top half of a double boiler, then remove from the heat. Pour in the herbal infusions and stir well. Grease a few cookie cutters (the kind that are open on both ends) with the vegetable oil, then seal some foil over the sharp edge of each cutter so that the foil acts like a false bottom. Rest foil side down on a cookie sheet. When the soapy infusion has cooled, add the rose hip, peppermint, and tea tree oils. Beat well with a whisk. Gently pour the mixture into the molds, then leave them to set for 24 hours in a cool, dark place. A refrigerator is ideal. When the soap has hardened, all you need to do is remove the foil and push through the molded soap. Wrap in waxed paper.

❦ *Betty's Victorian Citrus Balls*

A generations-old recipe for a delightful skin cleanser, these balls contain potent plant extracts that penetrate deep into the epidermis to cleanse and heal. Their natural exfoliant and humectant properties leave the skin baby soft and vibrantly toned.

1 cup soft vegetable glycerin soap (unscented, uncolored)

5 tablespoons medium-ground oatmeal

1 tablespoon finely grated citrus peel (orange, lemon, lime, or grapefruit—chose one per recipe)

2 tablespoons cold-pressed almond oil

5 drops lemon or lime or neroli essential oil (optional)

Finely grate the glycerin soap and place it in the top half of a double boiler. Heat until melted, but don't let it boil (keep a watchful eye). Remove from heat and stir in the oatmeal and the grated citrus peel. Continue stirring. Add the almond and the neroli oils, stirring after you add each. Once mixture is cool enough to touch, divide it into four equal parts, then roll each into a small ball. Place on a wire cooling rack to harden overnight. Wrap in tissue paper and store in a cool, dark place. Moisten skin with a skin nourishing infusion, such as the Rose Hip–Comfrey Mist (page 63), before cleansing with these citrus treats.

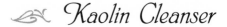

Kaolin Cleanser

This is an excellent cleanser for oily and combination complexions. Acne-prone skin will benefit from the deep-cleansing actions of this paste. Apply a thick layer and let it penetrate the skin while you relax. Nature does the healing for you!

1 tablespoon kaolin clay

1 tablespoon warm mineral water

2 teaspoons aloe gel

1 tablespoon oatmeal (finely ground)

5 drops lavender essential oil

In a small bowl, mix the kaolin with the warm water into a smooth paste. Add the aloe and stir. Sprinkle the oatmeal over the paste and combine. Add the lavender essential oil, one drop at a time, stirring the mixture after each drop is added.

Pin your hair off your face and forehead. Using a small sea sponge or your fingertips, evenly apply the paste to your face, layering it over your forehead, chin, and nose. Relax for 5 minutes. Rinse thoroughly, then apply a moisturizer.

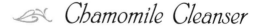 # Moisturizing Baby Cleanser

This gentle bar is soothing and nurturing. The ingredients are so mild that it can be used on babies' delicate skin without disrupting their sensitive pH balance.

 4 tablespoons chamomile flower infusion
 ½ cup soft vegetable glycerin soap
 2 teaspoons coconut oil
 1 teaspoon cold-pressed olive oil
 1 teaspoon lavender blossom honey
 5 drops geranium essential oil
 1 teaspoon vegetable oil (to grease molds)

Make the chamomile infusion by placing 2 tablespoons of fresh or 1 tablespoon dried chamomile flowers in 3 cups of very hot water. Cover and steep for 1 hour. Strain and set the infusion aside. Finely grate the glycerin soap. Place it in the top half of a double boiler. Heat until melted. Remove from the heat, add the infusion, and beat the mixture vigorously. Add the plant oils and honey and whip again. Add the geranium essential oil and stir the mixture after each drop is added. Grease a few soap molds or cookie cutters with the vegetable oil, and set them on a foil-lined baking sheet. Pour the scented mixture into the molds and leave to harden overnight. Then wrap in waxed paper to store.

Chamomile Cleanser

Generations of women have used almond oil and cocoa butter to soften dry skin and soothe irritated blemishes. This sweet-scented cleanser contains healing chamomile, protecting cocoa butter, and skin-softening almond oil. Together, they dissolve excess sebum and even remove stubborn waterproof mascara.

4 tablespoons cocoa butter

8 tablespoons sweet almond oil

10 drops chamomile essential oil

Place the cocoa butter in the top half of a double boiler and heat to gently melt. Remove from the heat, add the almond oil, and beat vigorously with a whisk. Once cooled, add the chamomile essential oil, one drop at a time, stirring the mixture after each drop is added.

Using your fingertips, dab small amounts of the chamomile cleanser onto your skin, then massage, using light, circular motions. Leave to penetrate for 5 minutes; then, using a cotton ball dipped in hot water, rinse a little off at a time. Repeat until all the cleanser has been removed. Rinse a washcloth in cold water, wring, then cover your face and relax for 10 minutes. Pat dry. Follow with a mist, such as the Burdock Facial Mist (page 63).

Skin Food Tonic and After-Bath Skin-Healing Dusting Powder

Barley and oats are good inside-out and outside-in skin foods. Either applied or eaten, both work to cleanse, nourish, and detoxify. Cooked oats and barley make a soothing wash water for treating dermatitis, psoriasis, eczema, sunburn, poison ivy, and dry skin. This tonic will make your skin feel soft and will speed up cell regeneration.

8 tablespoons rolled oats

8 tablespoons unhulled barley (or pearl)

4 cups mineral water

4 tablespoons fresh aloe gel

2 tablespoons slippery elm bark (powdered)

1 cup sage leaf infusion (see instructions for making infusions on page 36)

Place the oats and barley into a saucepan with the water and bring to a boil. Simmer for 15 minutes, then strain. Save cooked grains for a healthy breakfast; otherwise, discard them. Once liquid has cooled, add the aloe gel and slippery elm powder. Whisk briskly, then add the sage infusion. Run a warm bath, then pour in the Skin Food Tonic and let it disperse. Relax in the bath for 15–20 minutes.

AFTER-BATH SKIN-HEALING DUSTING POWDER

For those prone to outbursts of psoriasis, eczema, or other irritated skin conditions, apply this powder after bathing in the barley-oat Skin-Food Tonic. This healing powder quickly stops bleeding from open scrapes and cuts and helps dry up sores. Best of all, it doesn't sting, so it's ideal for children.

  8 tablespoons dried and powdered aloe leaf
  8 tablespoons dried and powdered slippery elm bark
  8 tablespoons dried and powdered comfrey root
  8 tablespoons dried and powdered goldenseal
  5 drops lavender essential oil
  3 drops tea tree essential oil

Combine all the ingredients and lightly whisk. Place the mixture into a shaker jar or powder puff box. After bathing, if you have any insect bites, skin blisters, itchy lesions, or rashes, sprinkle 1 teaspoon of slippery elm powder over the irritated skin (wet), and it will form a hard, protective scab over the wound. This recipe helped me and my three toddlers through chicken pox. The slippery elm "scab" was almost impossible to pick off.

The combination of the tonic bath and healing powder can be used twice daily. If the skin condition shows no improvement in 5–7 days, consult your dermatologist or physician.

Galen's Cold Cream Cleanser

I named this sweetly-scented cleanser after Galen, a Greek physician who developed the first cold cream during the second century. Rose water has been a favorite of generations of women, who combine it with other skin-softening ingredients to keep skin smooth and sweet-smelling all day. This cleanser safely moisturizes both aging and baby skin. It makes a wonderful diaper cream, hand lotion, and fragrant body moisturizer. Commercial cold creams contain mineral oil, used for its long shelf life, but this natural recipe uses only cold-pressed plant oils and lecithin, which easily penetrate the skin's surface.

> 2 tablespoons beeswax pearls
> 6 tablespoons sweet almond oil
> 3 tablespoons jojoba bean oil
> 2 tablespoons lecithin granules
> 3 tablespoons rose water
> 4 drops rose essential oil

Melt the beeswax in the top of a double boiler. Remove from the heat and add the almond and jojoba bean oils. Whisk gently, then cool. Add the lecithin granules and beat vigorously. Using an eyedropper, add the rose water and essential oil, stirring the mixture as each drop is added. Once it is beaten into a smooth paste, it is ready to use. Any leftovers can be stored in a sterilized, shallow glass jar and sealed. Store in a dark cupboard. Discard after 6 weeks.

To apply, rinse your skin with warm water, then pat dry. Using your fingertips, massage small amounts of the cleanser over your face and upper neck just before bedtime, leave on for 15 minutes, then splash with warm water and pat dry. Or apply as an all-over moisturizer after showering.

Jon's Fennel Skin Tonic

Everyone has a few laughter lines, but it doesn't hurt to treat them right! This wonderfully refreshing and skin-soothing tonic tightens and tones, reducing wrinkles on your face and upper neck. Honey is mildly antiseptic and acts as a humectant, trapping moisture droplets on the skin's surface. Fennel has a sweet licorice-like aroma, which I love. I mix up a batch on hot, humid days when my skin needs a refreshing treat.

2 tablespoons vodka
1 teaspoon lavender blossom honey
1 tablespoon fennel seeds
1 tablespoon fresh aloe gel

Place the vodka, honey, and fennel seeds into a shallow glass jar. Seal and shake vigorously. Place the jar in a warm, dark cupboard for 3 days. Strain by placing a coffee filter paper inside a mesh strainer and pour the liquid through. Discard the fennel seeds. Mash the aloe gel, then add it to the solution. Pour back into the jar and place back in the warm cupboard for another day. Moisten your face and neck with a facial mist, such as the Flower Water Splash (page 64) and let air-dry before applying the fennel tonic.

Herbal Oat Balls for Baby

These sweet little cleansing balls are ideal for bathing infants, children, and even adults. They are skin-soothing and work wonders calming active kids. Put them in the tub as you run the bath and rub them over the skin. I have used these delightful little balls on my children since they were babies. All the ingredients are edible, so there's no worry when junior grabs one to suck or bite.

2 cups finely ground oatmeal
2 tablespoons dried chamomile flowers (ground)
1 tablespoon dried milk
1 tablespoon dried calendula flowers (ground)
1 pair clean panty hose (without holes or ladders)

Place the dry ingredients into a bowl and combine well. Cut the panty part of the hose off, leaving the two legs. Check for holes and runs, then stuff a handful of the mixture into one of the legs. Pack loosely, then seal with a knot. Repeat until you have 3 or 4 balls, then do the other leg. Store the balls in a lidded plastic or tin container in your bathroom. Drop one bag in the tub as you run a bath. Allow the milks and sweet scents to disperse. Wash your skin with the balls as you would use a washcloth. There is no need to apply a moisturizer after bathing, as both the oatmeal and milk are naturally moisturizing to your skin.

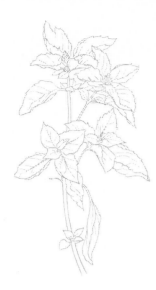

Scrubs and Packs

*S*crubs and deep-cleansing packs are wonderfully refreshing and invigorating ways of improving your skin's tone and texture. Massaging the skin with subtle, gritty substances clears away dead skin cells and excess sebum secretions, and it improves the overall appearance of the skin's surface. Both packs and scrubs can be applied to the skin with sea sponges, washing mitts, loofahs (but not the face), a rough washcloth, or your hands.

Your skin is the largest gland in your body. It flushes out wastes and accumulated toxins from millions of pores. This sophisticated system is easily affected by diet, so avoid refined foods and make sure that live proteins, vitamins, and minerals are part of your daily intake. Without them, collagen breaks down, and your skin may age prematurely. Keep your skin clear by treating it right from the inside and outside.

Skin brushing is another way to thoroughly cleanse the skin. It is one of the best ageless skin-beautifying techniques, and it has become part of my daily skin health ritual. The effectiveness of this technique of exfoliation can be measured by your skin's glow and soft texture. Dry-skin brushing encourages detoxification of the deeper dermal layers and promotes rapid lymphatic drainage. At the beginning and end of the day, I devote ten minutes to skin brushing with a chamomile and oat-milk splash wash, then air-dry until my skin tingles.

Exfoliation through brushing and the application of the following natural, living packs and scrubs will refresh, cleanse, and revitalize your skin. You need only glance at your reflection in the mirror after using a few of these recipes to know that your skin has been deeply nourished by these outside-in treatments.

Setting the Scene for a Full-Body Dry Skin Brush

This ageless beauty exercise stimulates and regenerates all skin tissues, inside and outside. It is remarkably detoxifying to the inner skin layers and eliminative organs. To reap its full benefits, brush your skin at least once a day.

Stand nude in a warm, well-ventilated room. Stretch your whole body from the tips of your toes to the top of your head to awaken your nerves. Sit in a comfortable position and begin stroking your skin with a natural-bristle brush. Begin at the balls of your feet and work your way up to the nape of your neck. Use sweeping stokes in an upward direction (toward the heart), being careful not to brush too hard over the soft skin of the breasts, abdomen, inner arms, thighs, and buttocks. Your skin will turn a light pink color and feel sensual and warm to the touch. Once your whole body has been brushed, take a warm shower, then finish off with 5–10 seconds of cold water. If privacy and weather permit, air-dry outside in the open air. If the sun is shining, this is an ideal opportunity to nourish your skin with rainbow light energy, promoting vitamin D absorption and awakening your inner energy centers.

Perform twice daily.

✑ Breast Tissue Scrub

*T*his delicately exfoliating scrub is remarkably toning to the soft breast tissue, encouraging elasticity and firmness. Almond meal can be purchased at any supermarket, but it is simple to grind at home from whole nuts in a coffee grinder.

    3 teaspoons sweet almond oil

    12 whole almonds with inner skins

    12 tablespoons medium-ground oatmeal

    2 tablespoons rose water

    1 teaspoon fresh aloe gel

Measure the almond oil into a small bowl. Grind the almonds (including their inner brown skins) in a coffee grinder or food processor. Add to the almond oil, then sprinkle the oatmeal over the oil and meal mixture. Whip together with the rose water. Last, add the aloe gel and stir. Mist your upper body with an herbal infusion, such as the rose hip infusion (page 36.) Then apply the scrub, massaging your breasts in small, circular movements. Leave for 10 minutes then rinse. Pat dry.

✑ Patricia's Acne Sage Pack

*S*age has earned its skin-nourishing reputation through generations of use. It is a powerful herb to be respected and used only in its dried or freshly picked form. It is an excellent skin regenerator. Here it cleanses and decongests toxic waste accumulations in the epidermal layers. I like to wet my skin with an herbal infusion, such as the Herb-Juice Wash (page 65) before applying this pack.

8 tablespoons strong sage leaf infusion

8 tablespoons fuller's earth

1 teaspoon aloe gel

Make the sage infusion (see instructions, page 36), and allow it to steep, covered, for 1 hour. Strain through a fine mesh. Pour into a bowl, then sprinkle in the fuller's earth. Whip vigorously with a whisk, then add the aloe gel and mix again into a smooth paste.

Massage the acne sage pack with sweeping motions, on to moist skin, especially the hard-to-reach area of your back, arms, neck, and face. Allow scrub to dry for 15 minutes, then rinse with tepid water. Air-dry and relax for 30 minutes.

﹋ *Alum Back Pack*

This is a deeply penetrating cleanser. Alum is a naturally occurring mineral that has astringent qualities. Tea tree essential oil heals wounds, stimulates the immune system, and soothes irritated skin. You will need some help applying this pack as most deeply embedded pimples, spots, and black-heads lurk menacingly in those hard-to-reach folds and creases in the middle of the back and around the shoulders. Unless you are a yoga expert, you'll need an assistant. Use an herbal mist, such as the Comfrey Elderflower Skin Mist (page 65) before applying.

3 teaspoons powdered sulfur (ask for it at your pharmacy)

1 tablespoon alum crystals

⅔ cup (100g) fuller's earth

2 egg whites, lightly beaten

6 drops tea tree essential oil

2 drops lavender essential oil

2 drops calendula essential oil

Combine the first 3 ingredients in a bowl. Fold in the beaten egg whites, and mix into a smooth paste. One drop at a time, add the tea tree, lavender, and calendula oils, stirring the mixture after each drop is added. Cover bowl with a cloth rinsed in cold water. Apply the pack to moistened skin and relax for 20 minutes. Rinse in a warm shower, then hydrate your skin by drinking 16 oz. of water.

✑ Knee and Elbow Scrub

Yogurt has been used as a simple cleanser for generations. It is conditioning and a delightful feast for the skin. Yogurt is rich in concentrated micronutrients, such as calcium. The oils are skin-soothing, and the honey, a gentle antiseptic, heals and tones.

1 tablespoon cold-pressed wheat germ oil

1 tablespoon cold-pressed apricot kernel oil

1 teaspoon aloe gel

½ teaspoon dandelion stalk juice

1 teaspoon flower blossom honey

1 tablespoon yogurt

2 teaspoons cornmeal

Place the wheat germ and apricot kernel oils into a small bowl with the aloe gel. Whip gently with a hand whisk. Extract the sticky, white fluid from at least 20 large dandelion flower stalks by cutting off the flower head and using a small eyedropper to suck the fluid out. Immediately add this volatile fluid to the oil and aloe mixture, then add the honey and yogurt. Whip again. Sprinkle the cornmeal over the sticky mix, then stir.

Apply scrub, leave for 10 minutes, then rinse.

✒ *Christina's Butter Scrub*

Another skin treat that smells as good as it looks, it is rich in potent plant oils and marine minerals that actively detoxify and tone. The almond oil softens dry skin and soothes blemishes. The combination of the crunchy nut butter and salt granules exfoliates and nourishes.

    2 tablespoons sweet almond oil
    1 teaspoon finely ground sea salt
    2 teaspoons finely ground kelp seaweed
    1 tablespoon aloe gel
    4 tablespoons crunchy whole-nut butter

Combine the ingredients in a small bowl and whip into a gritty paste.

Apply body butter scrub to your breasts, neck, and face, using your hands to massage it into your skin. Relax for 15 minutes, then rinse with warm water. Follow with Aromatic Vinegar Wash (page 66).

Dilly's Grit Scrub

This scrub is so simple and so nutritious, your skin will lap up its goodness and glow with good health for days.

4 tablespoons ground oatmeal

1 tablespoon fine sea salt

1 teaspoon granulated kelp

1 teaspoon brewer's yeast (3 crushed tablets)

2 tablespoons granulated brown sugar

1 tablespoon slippery elm bark (powdered)

Place all the ingredients into a sterilized, shallow glass jar and seal.

It's best to apply this scrub in the shower. Rinse, then turn off the water leaving your skin moistened. While standing in the warm steam take a handful of the oatmeal-grit body scrub and gently massage it into your skin. Cover every inch of skin you can reach. Leave for 5–10 minutes, then massage again as you rinse with warm water. Once all the scrub is removed, refresh your skin for a few seconds with a tepid shower. Wrap yourself in a warmed bath sheet, and relax.

Crystal's Upper Neck Pack

This deep-cleansing and surface-healing pack works wonders, tightening sagging tissues under the chin and around the neck. The honey and aloe are soothing and gently antiseptic, binding broken or stretched tissue, while the naturally astringent fresh potato and cucumber reduce puffiness. I like to moisten my skin with Orange Flower Refresher (page 67) before applying this pack.

½ cup fresh aloe gel

1 tablespoon fresh cucumber juice

1 medium-sized potato (grated, with skin)

1 tablespoon lavender blossom honey

Place the aloe gel in a bowl, then add the fresh cucumber juice. Whip gently with a hand whisk and set aside. Grate the unpeeled potato and add to the bowl. Stir well, then drizzle the honey over the mixture. Refrigerate for 5 minutes.

Apply to still moist, freshly showered skin. Using your hands, pile layers of the potato and aloe pack on your chin, neck, and shoulders. Lie down for 10 minutes and relax. Rinse off with warm water, pat dry, then apply a light moisturizer.

❧ Witch Hazel Deep Penetrating Pack

This simple cleansing scrub is gentle yet invigorating. It removes dead skin cells and embedded impurities from clogged pores. The floral vinegar splash (applied after the scrub), was particularly popular with Victorian women who used it as a tonic for their complexions. Vinegar restores the skin's natural acid balance. Together, these treatments are skin-nourishing, balancing, and exfoliating.

4 tablespoons almond meal

2 tablespoons finely ground oatmeal

1 teaspoon cornmeal

1 teaspoon brewer's yeast (3 crushed tablets)

1 tablespoon distilled witch hazel solution

1 tablespoon fresh aloe gel

2 tablespoons yogurt

Combine the first four ingredients in a bowl, then transfer into a sterilized, shallow glass jar and seal. For a single application, put 1 tablespoon of the dry mixture in a bowl with the witch hazel, aloe, and yogurt, and whip into a smooth paste.

Apply pack, using your hands, then relax for 10 minutes. Rinse off and dry. Follow with a splash, such as Lavender Vinegar Splash (page 67) then air-dry in a warm room.

Min's Cornmeal Thigh Scrub

This delightfully aromatic scrub works exfoliating wonders. The natural botanicals and cold-pressed oils work together to loosen stubborn cellulite and soften the surrounding skin. Massage your thighs twice a week for remarkable results.

1 small avocado stone

4 tablespoons cornmeal

2 teaspoons aloe gel

1 tablespoon cold-pressed grape seed oil

6 drops juniper essential oil

6 drops lemon essential oil

Put the avocado pit in heavy paper bag, then wrap the bag around the pit a few times. With a hammer or wooden mallet, give the pit a few good whacks to break it up into smaller pieces that will fit into a coffee grinder or small food processor. Grind the pieces to a gritty meal consistency. Mix with the cornmeal, then place in a sterilized shallow jar, seal, and label. Pour the aloe, grape seed, juniper, and lemon oils into a bowl, then sprinkle about 2 teaspoons of the avocado and cornmeal over the wet ingredients and stir. Add additional meal if necessary so that you have a gritty paste.

Beautiful Face, Beautiful Body

Mist your legs thoroughly (try the Ginseng Mist on page 67), then apply the paste, using small, circular, massaging motions. Relax for 15 minutes and rinse with warm water.

❧ *Strawberry Belly and Breast Scrub*

This is one of my favorite soft-skin body scrubs, and it smells as delicious as it feels. Fresh, ripe strawberries make an excellent skin cleanser and moisturizer. They are rich in healthy skin nutrients (such as vitamins A, C, and E) and possess a harmonious pH balance, like human skin itself.

> 12 ripe strawberries
>
> 2 tablespoons cold-pressed avocado oil
>
> 4 tablespoons pureed cucumber (with skin and seeds)
>
> 3 tablespoons distilled witch hazel solution
>
> 3 tablespoons rice flour
>
> 1 teaspoon aloe gel

Trim the strawberry stems, cut away any white parts, then mash with a fork. Pour the avocado oil into another bowl, add the pureed cucumber, and stir well. Add the mashed strawberries and witch hazel. Sprinkle the rice flour over the wet mixture and fold in. Last, add the aloe and stir to form a smooth paste.

Mist your breasts and upper chest (try the Orange-Lavender Mist on page 68) leave for 5 minutes, then apply the scrub with your hands or a sea sponge. Relax for 15 minutes, then rinse thoroughly. Dry and moisturize.

Bionutrient Mud Pack

I use this nutrient-packed skin treat just before heading off on a beach vacation, when I want my skin to look its best. Apple juice helps to firm the facial and upper neck tissues. Lemon juice has an age-old reputation for maintaining healthy and young-looking skin. This pack deeply cleans and invigorates gray, slack, or blotchy skin. I like to drench my skin from ankles to neck with Calendula Skin Spray (page 68) before using this pack.

2 tablespoons cold-pressed sweet almond oil

1 cup freshly extracted apple juice

8 tablespoons fuller's earth

1 tablespoon fresh lemon juice (not bottled)

1 tablespoon lavender flower honey

8 drops sandalwood essential oil

Measure the almond oil into a bowl, add the apple juice, and gently whisk. Sprinkle the fuller's earth and lemon juice over the mixture and stir. Drizzle over the honey, then add the essential oil, one drop at a time, stirring the mixture after each drop is added. Stir until you have a smooth paste.

Use your hands to apply the paste with swift, circular motions on your still-moistened skin. Run a hot shower for a few minutes. Turn off the water, then stand in the hot steam for 5 minutes. Rinse well, dry, and moisturize.

Aromatic and Therapeutic Baths

*U*tterly indulge yourself in a total bathing experience for a fraction of the cost you would pay at a European spa. Maybe you've heard of spas and clinics that are famous for their seaweed, enzyme, mustard, and mineral baths. You can treat yourself to all of them in your own home.

The skin is the largest organ of the body and does the all important work of absorbing moisture as well as nutrients. Baths are a wonderful part of a daily beauty regime. They not only relax the mind and spirit, they encourage both skin and cellular regeneration, increase energy levels, and decongest the skin. An herbal infusion of lavender, rosemary, chamomile, and sage, poured into a hot bath, will penetrate the deeper dermal layers, forcing out impurities and leaving the skin refreshed and cleaned.

My bathroom is my sanctuary. It is the only place in my home where I can lock the door and relax in a warm, soothing environment. I love soaking in an infusion of chamomile and lavender flowers and washing my skin with warmed oat milk in an aromatic, candlelit room. Bliss.

Beautiful Face, Beautiful Body

Joan's Rose Vinegar Bath

Skin-soothing and rich in vitamin C, this simple recipe relaxes me even after the most stressful day.

1 cup white wine vinegar
1 cup fresh pink rosebuds
½ cup fresh rose hips (crushed)
5 drops rose essential oil

Measure all the ingredients into a bowl and stir, then pour into a sterilized glass bottle, seal, and label with the contents and date. Place in a sunny window for 7–10 days. Shake the bottle daily to increase the process of dispersing the botanicals. Strain through a fine mesh. Add to a warm bath and soak for 20 minutes. To use in the shower, pour the rose vinegar bath on a washcloth and apply to freshly cleansed skin. Rinse. The vinegar can also be placed into a spray bottle and used as a refreshing after-bath mist.

Herbal Fizz Salt Bath

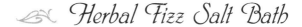

This simple therapeutic recipe does more than cleanse your skin, it heals and purifies even the deepest dermal layers. Take an herbal fizz bath twice a week. It's a refreshing way to cleanse clogged pores and balance sebaceous secretions.

½ cup baking soda
4 tablespoons cornstarch
2 drops wheat grass juice (pure chlorophyll)
3 tablespoons fresh lemon juice

5 drops of the following essential oils:

    Ylang ylang

    Calendula

    Chamomile

    Lemon

1 tablespoon cold-pressed sweet almond oil

Excluding the almond oil, combine all the ingredients in a bowl. The mixture will be dry as the juices and oils are quickly absorbed by the baking soda and cornstarch. Store in a sterilized, shallow glass jar and seal. Keep near the bathtub. Run a warm bath, pour in the almond oil, and swish it around the water with your hands to disperse. Sprinkle 1 tablespoon of the dry mixture into the bath. Soak for 20 minutes, then wrap yourself in a warmed bath sheet or blanket and rest for 15 minutes.

Claire's Herbal Bubble Bath

All bubble baths are fun and skin-tickling, especially for children. This recipe is so simple that, with a little supervision, even a child can make it. The carrot and beet root coloring and the lavender and chamomile fragrances are optional.

1 teaspoon of the following herbs:

    Rosemary leaves

    Lavender flowers

    Marigold flowers

    Peppermint leaves

    Rose petals

    Lemon balm leaves

    Chamomile flowers

2 tablespoons glycerin

2 tablespoons baby shampoo

1 tablespoon granulated sugar

    Optional:

    ¼ teaspoon carrot juice (natural yellow dye)

    ¼ teaspoon beet root juice (natural purple dye)

    2 drops lavender essential oil

    2 drops chamomile essential oil

Chop and crush the fresh herbs, then mix together and place in a shallow glass bottle. Measure 1 heaping tablespoon for this recipe. Make an infusion of the combined fresh herbs following the instructions on page 36. Cover and steep for 30 minutes, then strain. Pour the glycerin, shampoo, and herbal infusion into a large bowl, sprinkle the granulated sugar over the wet ingredients, and stir. Pour in the natural vegetable dyes and fragrances and mix again. Pour into a running bath and swish with your hands to disperse the potent botanicals and natural, skin-soothing cleansers. Immerse yourself and relax.

❧ Millie's Aromatic Mud Bath

Here is a deep-cleansing, pore-purifying experience for your whole body. The natural oils, herbs, and mud penetrate, detoxify, and promote cellular regeneration. Among the best home treatments, it intensively cleanses the whole body.

    2 teaspoons fresh marigold flowers

    2 teaspoons fresh lavender flowers

    2 teaspoons fresh pink rose petals

    1 cup very hot mineral water (for the infusion)

    1 tablespoon clear blossom honey

1 teaspoon yogurt

¼ cup kaolin clay

1 teaspoon powdered licorice root

10 drops neroli essential oil

½ cup fresh seawater (or 1 cup mineral water and 1 teaspoon sea salt)

Following the instructions on page 36, make the marigold, lavender, and rose flower infusion. Cover and steep for 30 minutes. Strain through a fine mesh. In a bowl, whip the honey and yogurt into a smooth paste. Add the kaolin, licorice root, and neroli essential oil and whisk vigorously. Run a very hot bath, turn off the water, then leave to cool. Add the seawater to the paste and whisk again. Apply the aromatic mud to your skin in a warm, steamy bathroom. Cover your whole body, from feet to face. Leave wide, clear-skin circles around your eyes and mouth. Test the bath water, adding cold if necessary, then immerse for 10 minutes. Rinse off with a cool shower.

❦ *Tina's Aromatic Bathing Crystals*

This is a simply delightful recipe to soothe tired, frazzled nerves. I find it especially rewarding after a demanding day in toddler world! It takes minutes to make and will last up to 6 months in a properly sealed container. These bathing crystals make excellent gifts.

1 cup coarse sea salt

5 drops chamomile essential oil

5 drops lavender essential oil

5 drops benzoin tincture

    Optional ingredients: 2 drops each of the following dyes

    Beet root juice

Carrot juice

Strawberry juice

Or wheat grass juice, alone

Measure sea salt into a bowl. Using an eyedropper, add the essential oils, benzion tincture, and natural vegetable dyes. Stir until the crystals take on an even, subtle scent and color. Transfer into a decorative glass bottle and keep near your bathtub. Sprinkle 2 heaping tablespoons in a warm bath. Swish bath water until the crystals have dissolved. Immerse and relax for 15–20 minutes.

Annha's Balsamic Toning Bath

This utterly skin-indulging bathing recipe uses some of the most potent botanical extracts available. They help the whole body relax and encourage cellular metabolism. Bathing just before bedtime in this tonic will induce a sound, restful sleep.

8 cups (2 quarts) mineral water

5 tablespoons organic rice flour

2 teaspoons of each of the following herbs:

Rosemary leaves

Pine buds (crushed)

Peppermint leaves

Juniper berries

Bay leaves

Marjoram leaves

Eucalyptus leaves

Silver birch

1 teaspoon dried and powdered aloe leaf

1 tablespoon powdered kelp

4 tablespoons kaolin clay

3 tablespoons cold-pressed sweet almond oil

Measure the water and rice flour into a large saucepan and bring to a boil. Remove from the heat and add the fresh herbs, aloe, and kelp. Cover and allow to steep for 30 minutes. Strain through a fine mesh, add the kaolin clay, and whisk vigorously. Pour the almond oil into a warm bath and stir the water with your hands. Add the infusion mixture and immerse yourself. Relax for 30 minutes.

Seabed Healing Bath

As a teenager, I developed psoriasis. Itchy, red, flaking lesions cropped up almost overnight. I was covered from head to foot. Quite unsightly! I was desperate to find a natural cure and discovered to my delight that swimming in the cold ocean worked wonders on my skin. With a little experimenting, I came up with this rich marine mineral paste. It both relieved the furious itching and reduced the size and color of the lesions. You can buy the seaweeds dried in most health food stores.

4 tablespoons fuller's earth

2 tablespoons dried and ground kelp seaweed

1 small piece fresh or hydrated laver seaweed (*Porphyra umbiliculis*)

2 teaspoons fresh or hydrated dulse seaweed

3 tablespoons fresh aloe gel

1 cup fresh seawater (or 1 cup water with 1 teaspoon sea salt)

1 tablespoon sweet almond oil

2 tablespoons chickweed infused oil

Beautiful Face, Beautiful Body

Mix the fuller's earth and kelp together. Chop the laver and dulse seaweeds finely and add them to the kelp mixture with the aloe gel and seawater. Stir to form a smooth, slippery paste. Standing in your tub or shower, apply the paste to your itchy and flaking skin using your hands or an old makeup brush. Leave it on for 10 minutes. Run a warm bath, add 1 tablespoon sweet almond oil to the water (to prevent your skin from drying), then immerse yourself and relax for a few minutes. Rinse in a warm spray, finishing off with a few cold splashes.

Apply the chickweed infused oil to your skin after bathing to promote cellular regeneration, draw out impurities, and relieve itching.

🙠 *Herbal After-Bath Body Powder*

This simple herbal powder contains natural herbal deodorizers. It keeps the skin refreshed and smelling sweet while you exercise. Arrowroot is strongly absorbent, and slippery elm bark is skin-soothing and healing.

- 1 teaspoon whole clove (ground into a powder)
- 1 teaspoon powdered slippery elm bark
- 2 teaspoons dried and ground orange peel
- ½ cup powdered arrowroot
- ½ cup baking soda
- ½ cup cornstarch

If you can't buy the clove, slippery elm, and orange peel in powdered form, grind it in a coffee grinder or food processor. Measure all the ingredients into a shallow glass jar and shake vigorously. Place in a dark cupboard for 2 weeks, shaking the contents daily. Use on dry skin daily after a bath or shower, or use as a natural deodorant.

1 tablespoon of the following powdered ingredients:

    Baking soda

    Slippery elm bark

    Cornstarch

    Arrowroot

    Goldenseal

    Comfrey root

Combine dry ingredients and place into a shallow glass jar. Seal and label with contents and date. Use on baby after diapering or bathing. This recipe is also ideal for people who prefer unscented bath products.

❧ Purifying Body-Balance Seaweed Bath

This toning, harmonizing, and skin-energizing bath works because the electrolyte magnetic actions of seaweed aid the release of body fluids from congested tissues and cells. Seaweeds dissolve accumulated fatty wastes so that they can be eliminated through the skin, and they replenish iron and potassium levels, helping to maintain hormonal and pH balances for ageless, beautiful skin. Collect the living ingredients fresh, if possible, or purchase them dried.

1 tablespoon kelp (*Laminaria digitata*) seaweed

1 tablespoon dulse (*Rhodymenia palmata*)

1 tablespoon sea lettuce (*Ulva lactuca*)

2 tablespoons Iceland moss (*Cetraria islandica*)

1 tablespoon dabberlocks (*Alaria esculenta*)

1 tablespoon dead sea salt

1 quart fresh seawater (or 1 quart water with 1 teaspoon sea salt)

2 teaspoons cold-pressed jojoba bean oil

Hydrate the dried seaweeds by placing them in a bowl of cold water. Leave for 15 minutes. Remove from the water, then chop finely. Place seaweeds in a bowl, then add the dead sea salt and seawater. Stir well. Before you begin your bath, light small, scented candles. Put on some soothing music. Place the seaweed into a bathtub, cover with hot water, then add cold so that when you immerse yourself, it feels cozy warm, not scorching hot or tepid. Pour the jojoba oil (to prevent your skin from drying) in the bathwater, and swish it around with your hands. Stay in the bath for 30 minutes to an hour, adding more hot water, if necessary. Towel off (or air-dry in the sunshine), then wrap yourself in a warm bathing sheet and relax.

✎ *Charming Your Skin with an Oxygen Bath*

This skin-energizing and rejuvenating bath is one of my favorites. On those days when I feel stressed or overtired, this tingling bathing tonic lifts my spirits. It is called an oxygen bath because the herbs cause an internal and external detoxification of the body, especially the lungs and skin.

1 tablespoon mullein leaves

1 tablespoon rosemary leaves

1 tablespoon eucalyptus leaves

1 tablespoon peppermint leaves

Loosely pack the herbs in a self-sealing tea bag or muslin cloth and seal with a rubber band. Drop the bag into a steaming-hot bath and leave for 15 minutes. Darken the room and light one scented candle or some incense. Put on some soothing music, and immerse your tired body for 30 minutes. Wash your skin with the herbal bag and breathe in the lung-clearing aromas.

⚁ *Hannba's Slimming Bath*

The woman who gave me this recipe claims it took inches off her waist! I won't vouch for that, but it does detoxify through the largest organ of the body: the skin. Make sure that you replenish your lost fluids by drinking a large glass of water when you get out.

> 3 tablespoons mustard seeds
> 3 tablespoons Epsom salts
> 1 teaspoon rosemary leaves (freshly crushed)
> ¼ cup plantain infused oil

Run a very hot bath, sprinkle the mustard seeds, Epsom salts, and rosemary leaves into the water. Close the door and allow the room to fill with the warm, aromatic steam for 15–20 minutes. Test the water before stepping in, adding more cold if necessary; you want to sweat, not cook! Immerse yourself for 20 minutes and let nature shed the pounds or inches. After drying yourself off, massage your skin with the plantain infused oil, using sweeping, upward motions. Wrap yourself in a warm bath sheet or blanket and relax. Drink at least one 12-oz. glass of mineral water to replenish your system before going to sleep.

⚁ *Luxury Milk Sunshine Bath*

I love the idea of bathing outside in the morning sunshine. These delightful fragrances and delicate cleansing milk will make you feel as though you have been transported to some exotic climate where bathing outside is commonplace. Indulge yourself twice a week, and experience an ageless, beautiful skin suit.

Beautiful Face, Beautiful Body

2 unscented oat-bag balls

2 cups chamomile infusion

3 tablespoons acacia honey

6–8 drops benzoin tincture

5 drops neroli essential oil

5 drops cinnamon essential oil

2 drops clove essential oil

1 quart whole-cream goat's milk (fresh, if possible)

2 tablespoons cold-pressed sweet almond oil

See page 96 for instructions to make the oat-bag balls. Make the chamomile infusion following the instructions on page 36. Steep the chamomile for 15 minutes, then strain it and drop the oat balls into the hot chamomile infusion. Leave for 10 minutes. Meanwhile, measure the honey and benzion tincture into a small bowl and beat gently. Add the essential oils. Squeeze the oat milk from each ball and pour the creamy infusion into a larger bowl. Add the goat's milk and the honey paste. Whisk vigorously. Run a warm bath, pour in the almond oil and disperse it with your hands. Pour the aromatic, milky solution into the bathwater. Immerse yourself and relax. Imagine you're in a sunny meadow: feel the healing sun on your skin as you wash your body with this delightful bathing milk.

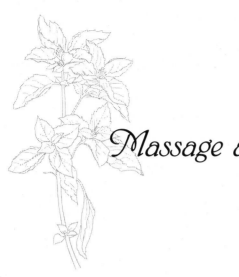

Massage and Body Oils

*M*assage is an art anyone can master. It is the most pleasurable, luxurious treatment for aches and pains. It is also used to treat headaches, nervous tension, stress, and some forms of depression. All forms of massage are effective at boosting blood circulation to the skin's surface, stimulating lymphatic drainage, and reducing cellulite. Best of all, it's a sensual treat for your partner anytime. Don't limit yourself to commercially available oils. It's easy to make your own massage blends, and you can tailor them to suit your personal needs and tastes.

✐ *Setting the Scene for a Relaxing Massage*

In a warm, well-ventilated room, scatter some pillows on the floor. Light a scented candle or burn a stick of incense. Put on some enchanting rainforest music or rhythmic ocean sounds or any soothing, sensual music. Warm your choice of oil. If you're the lucky partner on the receiving end of this massage, undress, then wrap a towel loosely over your lower back and legs. Lie down and get comfortable.

If you're giving the massage, pour a small amount of the warmed oil over your hands and rub them together. To completely massage the face, neck, and upper back, your partner can either lie on her back or sit in a comfortable (spine erect) position. The yoga lotus position is ideal for this part of the massage. Begin with your partner's face. Use small, circular motions and gently massage the forehead, temples, cheeks, nose, chin, and upper neck. Take your time. Massage the nape of neck and ears. With larger, sweeping strokes, move down the shoulders and then the back. Using more oil as necessary, turn your attention to the shoulders, arms, hands, and fingers. Apply more oil and move down the lower back, buttocks, and upper legs. Use sweeping strokes with light pressure. Move the towel to cover the top half of your partner's body while you concentrate on the legs, ankles, and feet. Pay special attention to the balls of the feet and each toe. Have your partner roll over onto her belly, then conclude with a fingertip massage over the shoulders, back, and bottom. Then, before leaving her to fall into a restful sleep, crack an imaginary egg on her crown and let the yolk slip down over her head and shoulders. Ah! Luxury.

Jo's Cellulite-Free Oil

This irresistible anticellulite formula is extraordinarily effective at breaking down the clumps of familiar fatty acid deposits, commonly referred to as cellulite. Used daily, morning and evening, you'll soon begin to see the dimpled skin improve in appearance.

> 4 tablespoons cold-pressed grape seed oil
>
> 2 teaspoons cold-pressed wheat germ oil
>
> 1 teaspoon fresh aloe gel
>
> 5 drops fennel essential oil
>
> 10 drops juniper berry essential oil
>
> 5 drops lemon essential oil

Measure the cold-pressed oils in a bowl, then stir in the aloe. Add the essential oils one drop at a time, stirring the mixture after each drop is added. Pour into a small, shallow jar, and seal.

To apply, warm your hands either by clapping five times or by washing them in hot water, then drying them. (Be sure your hands are dry before you begin.) Massage the oil into your legs and buttocks with sweeping, upward motions until it is thoroughly absorbed. Run a hot shower for 1 minute. Turn off the water, then step into the hot steam and continue massaging. Mist with 1 cup of chilled, sparkling mineral water. Wait 5 minutes, then wrap in a warm blanket and rest.

～ Relaxing Massage Oil and Herbal Hot Soak

Any cold-pressed oil infused with living, herbal extracts makes an outstanding massage treatment. Not only are they aromatically potent, they also promote toned skin. The following recipe includes herbs that relax the mind and body in unison.

4 tablespoons each of the following macerated plant oils:

> Chamomile
>
> Clary sage
>
> Basil
>
> Lavender
>
> Jasmine

5 drops chamomile essential oil

5 drops lavender essential oil

HERBAL HOT SOAK

1 cup lavender and chamomile flower infusion

1 cup rosemary leaf infusion

Make the chamomile, lavender, and rosemary infusions by following the instructions on page 36. Cover and steep for 1 hour. Funnel the macerated oils into a small bottle, then add the essential oils one drop at a time, shaking the bottle as each drop is added. Run a warm bath. Pour the rosemary (skin-oxygenating) and chamomile and lavender (healing and relaxing) infusions into the water. Immerse yourself for 15 minutes. Massage your skin from feet to neck, using the aromatic herbal massage oil, then wrap yourself in a warm blanket and put your feet up!

✑ Fragile Tissue Oil

This sensuous and nutritious oil works wonders on those laughter lines, drooping eyelids, and crow's-feet. Apricots are renowned for their cosmetic properties. Their high concentrations of antioxidant beta-carotene tone and refresh. Cinnamon adds its warm aroma to this mist and stimulates the skin. Note that it takes 2–3 weeks to make the pure carrot oil.

> 8 spring carrots (bright orange)
> ¼ cup cold-pressed sweet almond oil
> ½ cup cold-pressed apricot kernel oil
> 5 drops cinnamon essential oil

Grate the carrots, then place them in a shallow glass jar with a cork stopper. Fill to the very top with almond oil, then seal. Place the jar in a warm, dark place for 2–3 weeks. Strain through a fine mesh, then a paper coffee filter, squeezing out all the precious oil. (You'll only end up with about 1 tablespoon of carrot oil.) Funnel the apricot kernel, carrot, and cinnamon oils into a sterilized glass bottle, seal, date, and label. Keep out of sunlight and discard after 1 month.

Moisten your face with an herbal mist (such as Plantain Skin Mist page 69), then dab small amounts of the oil around your mouth and eyes and gently massage. Use nightly.

✑ Denise's Body Moisturizing Oil

This delicate, skin-enriching massage oil can be used as a moisturizer after showering or for toning the skin after a long soak in an herbal infusion bath. It is especially beneficial when massaged over chapped, cracked, and flaking skin.

1 teaspoon watercress juice

1 tablespoon cold-pressed wheat germ oil

4 tablespoons cold-pressed sweet almond oil

1 tablespoon cold-pressed avocado oil

10 drops geranium essential oil

2 tablespoons fresh aloe gel

Using a juicer, extract the fresh juice from the watercress (or place 5 sprigs of fresh watercress in a blender with ½ cup of mineral water, blend on high for 30 seconds, then strain). Soak a cotton ball into the juice, then dab it over your just-cleansed face. Leave to penetrate for 10 minutes (while you make up the rest of the recipe).

Measure the oils and aloe into a bowl and whisk together gently.

Rinse the skin-enriching watercress juice off your face. Run a hot shower for 5 minutes, turn off the water, then step into the shower and cover your body with the moisturizing oil. Massage it into your skin vigorously with sweeping, upward motions. Leave on overnight.

Adrian's Athlete's Muscle Oil

A wonderfully aromatic tonic for tired muscles, the essential oils soothe and regenerate tissues. Take it with you to the gym or use it at home after a run.

1 teaspoon shea butter

1 teaspoon cold-pressed wheat germ oil

6 tablespoons cold-pressed grape seed oil

1 teaspoon fresh aloe gel

5 drops lavender essesntial oil

5 drops mandarin essential oil

10 drops rosemary essential oil

Measure the shea butter, wheat germ oil, and grape seed oil into the top of a double boiler. Heat, stirring occasionally, until ingredients have blended. Remove from the heat, cover, and set aside. Combine the aloe and essential oils in a bowl, then stir into the oil mixture.

To apply: After exercising, first take a warm shower and dry yourself. Warm your hands by washing them in hot water, then dry them, and apply the oil to your legs using a petrissage (kneading) movement. The kneading lifts, presses, and rolls muscle tissue away from the bone to increase blood and lymphatic circulation, which detoxifies the muscles. Start out gently, then work the muscles harder, warming and flexing the skin. Leave the oil on to absorb into the skin.

Caution: Do not use this oil if you are pregnant. Rosemary essential oil is powerful and can trigger early uterine contractions and even induce premature labor.

Orange Flower Moisturizing Oil

Sensuous, romantic, and richly nourishing, this body lotion deeply moisturizes with the irresistible charm of oranges and roses. Used after bathing, it locks moisture to the skin's surface and leaves it feeling silky-soft and refreshed.

1 tablespoon borax powder

5 tablespoons rose water

2 tablespoons cold-pressed olive oil

3 drops cinnamon essential oil

3 drops neroli essential oil

2 drops ylang ylang essential oil

5 tablespoons orange flower water

Place the borax and rose water in the top half of a double boiler and heat through. Stir the mixture until all traces of powder have dissolved. Warm the olive oil by placing it in a small bowl, inside a saucepan half filled with hot water. Then blend into the rose water mixture. Add the essential oils, one drop at a time, stirring the mixture after each drop is added. Last, pour in the orange flower water and whisk gently.

After bathing or showering, apply to wet skin with sweeping, upward motions, covering your skin from head to toe.

Muscle-Relaxing Massage Oil

This highly aromatic and deep-muscle massage oil is made from an infusion of fresh herbs, spices, and essential oils. Use after a hard workout.

1 teaspoon of the following herbs:

> Cinnamon bark (finely ground)
>
> Verbena leaves
>
> Whole cloves (crushed)
>
> Marjoram leaves
>
> Chamomile flowers
>
> Rosemary leaves
>
> Sage leaves
>
> Thyme leaves

½ teaspoon mace

3 cups brandy

1 tablespoon horsetail herb (crushed)

1 cup cold-pressed grape seed oil

10 drops lemon essential oil

Place all the herbs (excluding the horsetail), and mace into a bottle and cover with the brandy. Seal and label and steep for 2 weeks, shaking the contents daily. Strain through a fine mesh. Make a decoction of the horsetail herb (follow instructions for making a herbal decoction, page 39), then cool and strain. Pour both liquids into a bowl. Add the grape seed oil, then whip vigorously. Last, drop in the lemon essential oil and stir. After soaking in a hot bath for 15–20 minutes, dry off and massage the oil into your legs, arms, upper chest, and abdomen.

Caution: Do not use while pregnant.

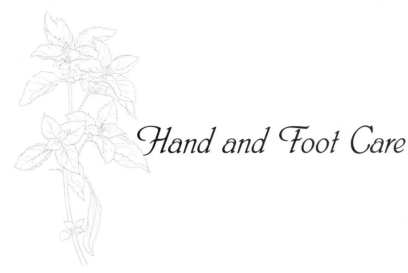

Hand and Foot Care

*Y*our hardworking extremities are often the most neglected parts of your body. Hands and feet need occasional pampering, too. The protective skin on your feet and hands is much thicker than the skin covering other parts of your body. Layers of hard, rough skin can sometimes become chapped and split. It's not just unsightly, it can also be very painful. Your hands are continually exposed to harsh weather from biting wind, heavy rain, and intense summer sunshine. Strong sunlight encourages the development of brown (or white) pigmentations, known as age spots. The bitter cold wind and rain can split and irritate already-sore skin.

Your fingernails and toenails need tender loving care to keep them strong and healthy, too. The best source of absorbable protein for beautiful hands and feet is obtained from plant foods. Fingernails grow about 1 cm. each week (twice as fast as toenails). It takes about 3 months for a fingernail to grow out completely. Beautiful nails need vitamins A and C, good circulation, and plenty of mineral-rich building blocks.

Your feet bear the brunt of another form of stress: your body weight. Don't squash your feet into tight boots, high heels, or synthetic running shoes (which suffocate and increase pungent foot odors). Over time, you'll pay the price in blisters and calluses. During the winter months, feet are prone to yet another stressor: suffocation. Socks, heavy blankets, woolly stockings, and tights prevent beautiful feet from breathing. Happy feet make happy faces. I can tell when my children's feet are unhappy by the expressions they wear on their faces. With a small amount of pampering your pinkies, you'll wear a smile on your face all year round.

Almond Cuticle Cream

This excellent nail-nourishing cream is rich in essential oils known to heal minor skin irritations and prevent the development of fungal nail infections. It also encourages and improves nail growth and texture. Your nails will begin to look more elegant and shapely from the easily absorbed micronutrients in this delightful cream.

    1 teaspoon beeswax pearls
    4 tablespoons cold-pressed sweet almond oil
    2 teaspoons fresh aloe gel
    5 drops lavender essential oil
    5 drops tea tree essential oil

Measure the beeswax into the top half of a double boiler and heat until it melts. Remove from the heat, then add the almond oil and whisk. Cool, then add the aloe gel and essential oils. Whisk once more. Massage into cuticles and hard nail surfaces daily.

Sonja's Fungal Foot Bath

This pungent foot bath treats infections of the toes, heels, balls, and ankles. It is deeply cleansing and invigorating to tired, sore, or swollen feet that have been stuffed into thick socks or pinching shoes. The skin-nutritious foot bath is also an excellent treat for those tootsies overworked by running, skiing, or dancing.

POWDER:

2 teaspoons powdered arrowroot

4 crushed juniper berries

INFUSION:

1 small (finely chopped) onion

$\frac{3}{8}$-inch-thick gingerroot (crushed)

2 small garlic cloves (crushed)

1 tablespoon fresh sage leaves

1 tablespoon fresh rosemary leaves

1 gallon very hot (not boiling) water

OTHER INGREDIENTS:

10 drops tea tree essential oil

10 drops lavender essential oil

1 tablespoon sweet almond oil

Infuse the powdered arrowroot with the juniper berries by crushing the tiny berries and covering them with the arrowroot. Place in a sterilized, sealed container for 2 weeks. After this period, sieve out the berries and rebottle. Make the pungent infusion by immersing the first five ingredients in the hot water. Cover, and steep for 30 minutes. Strain through a fine mesh, then pour into a foot bath. Add the tea tree and lavender oils and use your hands to stir. Then add the almond oil, immerse your feet, and relax. Make sure that you thoroughly dry your feet after soaking, especially between your toes. Dust feet with the arrowroot powder after soaking.

❧ Hard Skin Soothing Oil

This overnight intensive treatment locks moisture into hard skin surfaces. Seal this rapidly penetrating oil into the skin with cotton gloves or socks. The body's natural heat will encourage deeper penetration.

    3 tablespoons cold-pressed sweet almond oil

    1 tablespoon cold-pressed wheat germ oil

    1 teaspoon evening primrose oil

    5 drops benzoin tincture

    5 drops lavender essential oil

    5 drops mandarin esential oil

Place the first three ingredients into the top half of a double boiler to warm through. Remove from the heat and cool. Add the benzoin tincture and essential oils, one drop at a time, stirring the mixture after each drop is added. Wash your feet and hands, then dry them. Apply lavish quantities of the soothing oil to your hands and feet, then cover with cotton gloves and/or socks. Leave on overnight.

❧ Gabrielle's Sage Foot Powder

This sensual recipe is for tired, neglected feet that are crying out for attention. Put a generous dusting in your shoes or apply lavishly to bare, clean feet. Then put your feet up and relax. You'll feel a difference immediately.

    2 tablespoons fresh elder leaves

    2 tablespoons sage leaves

    1 tablespoon club moss spores

1 tablespoon slippery elm bark (powdered)

2 tablespoons rice flour

½ cup kaolin clay

2 tablespoons baking soda

2 tablespoons arrowroot powder

5 drops (each) of the following essential oils:

    Peppermint

    Thyme

    Lemon

    Clary sage

Using a mortar and pestle or a food processor, grind the first four ingredients, then place in a large bowl. Add the remaining ingredients, leaving the essential oils for last. Filter through a fine mesh, removing any sharp pieces of plant matter, and place into a shaker jar. Shake container well before each use. Dust shoes and socks before you put them on in the morning, and dust feet daily after bathing.

Lecithin Cuticle Lotion and Mullein Vinegar Soak

This nail-nourishing lotion can be applied as a manicure treatment to cleanse and moisturize the fingertips and nails.

2 teaspoons lanolin

1 teaspoon fresh aloe gel

1 tablespoon lecithin granules

5 drops clary sage esential oil

Measure the ingredients into a small bowl and whisk into a smooth paste.

VINEGAR SOAK

1 teaspoon vegetable glycerin

1 teaspoon fresh mullein flowers (crushed)

1 teaspoon white wine vinegar

2 tablespoons sweet almond oil

1 teaspoon rose water

Measure all the ingredients into a bowl and whisk well. Let stand for 5 minutes. Apply soak to hands and allow to penetrate for 15 minutes. Rinse and dry. Apply by massaging the lotion into cuticles daily, just before bed. Wear clean cotton gloves to bed to trap precious moisture.

Cocoa Butter Hand Barrier Cream

This waterproof cream acts as a moisture barrier. It heals and aids cellular regeneration, protecting the skin's surface from harsh environmental stressors. The lavender essential oil is said to increase the rate of healing, binding wounds quickly and soothing irritated blemishes. It lends its antiseptic and sebum-balancing properties to this delightful, aromatic hand cream.

3 tablespoons cocoa butter

3 tablespoons cold-pressed sweet almond oil

1 tablespoon cold-pressed castor oil

2 teaspoons beeswax pearls

5 drops geranium essential oil

5 drops lavender essential oil

Place the cocoa butter, almond and castor oils, and beeswax into the top half of a double boiler. Heat, stirring occasionally, until the cocoa butter and beeswax are melted and the ingredients have thoroughly blended. Remove from the heat and cool. Add the essential oils and beat vigorously. Using your fingertips, rub small amounts of the cream into your hands and nails. A great gift for gardeners!

✌ Almond Hand Paste

A simple soap alternative.

    10 whole almonds (with skins)
    4 tablespoons brandy
    1 tablespoon fresh lemon juice
    1 tablespoon cold-pressed sweet almond oil
    1 tablespoon fresh aloe gel
    3 drops benzoin tincture

Grind the almonds into a fine meal using a small food processor or coffee grinder. Mix with the other ingredients and knead into a ball. Place in plastic wrap and refrigerate for 30 minutes. Pinch off a bit of the paste, add warm water, and massage into your hands to exfoliate the skin and buff the nails. Use daily. If stored in an airtight container, the paste will remain potent for 2–3 weeks.

✌ Sam's Protein-Enriched Nail Food

This nourishing nail oil leaves the surrounding skin soft and supple. The salt is exfoliating, the honey antiseptic, and the wheat germ oil soothing and skin-purifying. Egg yolks contain moisture-locking lecithin, and the aloe is skin-binding and softening.

1 egg yolk

1 teaspoon sea salt

1 tablespoon cold-pressed castor oil

1 teaspoon cold-pressed wheat germ oil

1 teaspoon honey

3 drops benzoin tincture

1 tablespoon rose water

Measure all the ingredients into a small bowl and whip gently with a whisk. Pour into a sterilized, shallow glass jar and keep in the bathroom for daily use. Using a damp cotton swab, apply 2–3 coats of this nail food to each fingernail and toenail. Allow to completely dry, then reapply.

⟡ *Hard Skin Buffing Cream*

Ideal for buffing away calluses on the palms of the hands and balls of the feet, this cream heals, soothes, and moisturizes chapped, flaking skin on elbows, knuckles, and knees.

3 tablespoons cocoa butter

2 tablespoons cornmeal

1 tablespoon fuller's earth

1 tablespoon fresh aloe gel

5 drops mandarin essential oil

5 drops lemon essential oil

Measure the cocoa butter into the top half of a double boiler. Heat through, then remove from the heat and add the cornmeal and fuller's earth. Mix into a smooth paste. Add the aloe and essential oils, then stir again. Wash your hands in warm water, then dry them. Massage cream gently into hard skin. Leave on for 20 minutes, then rinse off.

A scrumptious aromatic cream to use after a soak in the tub, this is especially soothing for swollen, overworked feet, strained ankles, and pouting calves. Use daily as a natural foot treat.

1 tablespoon beeswax pearls

1 tablespoon cocoa butter

2 teaspoons wine tincture of catechu (see appendix for mail order suppliers)

30 drops propolis (resin) tincture

3 teaspoons kaolin clay

1 teaspoon rice flour

2 teaspoons of the following infused herbal oils:

> Marigold
>
> Lavender
>
> Rosemary
>
> Sage

1 teaspoon dried bay leaves (crushed)

½ cup mineral water

20 drops lavender essential oil

Melt the beeswax and cocoa butter in the top half of a double boiler. Measure the catechu and propolis tincture into a bowl with the kaolin clay, rice flour, and herbal oils. Rest the bowl inside a saucepan of hot water and beat thoroughly into a smooth paste. Make an infusion with the bay leaves and the mineral water. Steep for 15 minutes, strain, and cool. Stir into the paste and add the lavender essential oil, one drop at a time, stirring the mixture after each drop is added.

Bathe and dry feet thoroughly. Massage the cream into your feet, ankles, and calves at the end of the day.

Palm and Ball Washing Granules

*H*ere's an easy-living cleansing formula for your hands and feet. It can be made within minutes and used immediately or stored for up to 1 month. It takes up only a little space in your makeup bag, so it's a great treat for travelers.

4 tablespoons fresh whole almonds (ground finely)

1 tablespoon powdered orrisroot

1 tablespoon rice flour

2 tablespoons dried aloe leaf (ground finely)

5 drops lavender essential oil

5 drops neroli essential oil

3 drops tea tree essential oil

2 drops jasmine essential oil

Measure the first 4 dry ingredients in a bowl, then add the essential oils, one drop at a time, stirring the mixture after each drop is added. Dampen your hands and work the granules over rough skin for a few minutes, then rinse with warm water. Store excess in a sterilized, dark-colored glass bottle. Seal and label with contents and date.

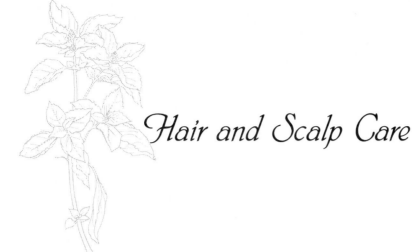

Hair and Scalp Care

*Y*our hair should be your crowning glory. You can coax lifeless hair back to lustrous health with the homemade herbal and fruit treatments on the following pages. Hair follicles are moistened by natural sebum secretions from the glands in the scalp. This oil travels along each strand of hair, coating and protecting it. There are many factors that hinder the natural vitality of your scalp. Poor diet is one. Foods rich in the vitamin B complex and vitamins A and C are the most important hair nutrients. The essential fatty acids and zinc also contribute to a head of shiny hair. A zinc-poor diet slows down hair growth and may even stop it altogether. Preventable environmental factors such as smoking, alcohol, stress, dehydration, and harsh chemical shampoos and conditioners all conspire to ruin the condition and texture of your hair.

Over time, washing with detergent-based shampoos, using electric dryers and curlers, and brushing with a nylon-bristle brush will reduce your lustrous hair to a tangled mass of unruly curls or frizz. All hair types benefit from conditioning treatments that protect the hair follicles and encourage growth. Massaging these treatments into the hair feeds malnourished hair follicles and stimulates circulation in the scalp. Dry and chemically damaged hair should be treated to an intensive moisturizing preparation once a week.

Rum After-Shampoo Conditioner

A delightful-smelling conditioner that is gentle and follicle-nourishing, it is especially recommended for the blonds among us.

    1 egg yolk
    4 tablespoons dark rum
    1 teaspoon aloe gel
    1 teaspoon cold-pressed avocado oil

Lightly whip the egg yolk, adding the rum a little at a time until used up. Add the aloe and avocado oil, then whip again. Shampoo, rinse thoroughly, then apply this conditioner. Massage deeply into the scalp and leave it on for 15 minutes. Rinse with tepid water and air-dry your hair.

DIETARY HELP: SESAME AND NETTLE TEA

    3 teaspoons sesame seeds
    1 cup water
    1 tablespoon nettle infusion

Dried nettles can be purchased from all good health food stores (but I like to pick them fresh from my garden). Measure the sesame seeds into a saucepan with the water. Bring to a boil. Simmer for 20 minutes, then strain and cool. Place 5 sprigs of fresh nettle leaves (or 1 tablespoon of dried) into a saucepan with 2 cups of mineral water. Cook until tender. Strain the herb and eat it like spinach, and save the cooking juice. Combine the sesame tea and nettle infusion and set aside to cool. Drink twice daily to bring back the natural color and shine to your hair.

Mint-Aloe Scalp Lotion and Vinegar Rinse

This unusual clay-based treatment removes dead skin cells from the scalp and absorbs excess sebum secretions. All the ingredients are deeply penetrating, nourishing even the deeper dermal tissues.

8 tablespoons coconut oil

4 tablespoons fuller's earth

½ cup chamomile infusion

2 tablespoons cider vinegar

1 tablespoon fresh aloe gel

10 drops peppermint essential oil

Heat the coconut oil in the top half of a double boiler on low. Remove from the heat, then sprinkle the fuller's earth over the oil. Whisk to form a paste and set aside. Make the chamomile infusion following the instructions on page 36. Cover and steep for 30 minutes, then strain through a fine mesh. Mix ½ cup of the infusion with a paste and cider vinegar, then whip again. Once cool, add the peppermint essential oil.

Part hair in rows and apply with a soft brush to the scalp. Leave on for 15 minutes, then rinse.

VINEGAR RINSE

FOR FAIR HAIR	FOR DARK HAIR
1 tablespoon chamomile infusion	1 tablespoon sage infusion
½ cup vinegar	½ cup vinegar
½ cup water	½ cup water

Make the chamomile or sage infusion following the instructions on page 36. Measure off 1 tablespoon, then add the other ingredients. Do a strand test (see page 164). Leave on your hair for 15 minutes, then rinse with tepid water until it runs clear. Allow your hair to air-dry.

Sandalwood Shampoo and Mineral-Rich Rinse

This delightful aromatic shampoo is gentle on the scalp.

2 tablespoons soapwort root (chopped)

1 teaspoon gingerroot (crushed)

3 tablespoons fresh chamomile flowers

1 cup very hot (not boiling) water

1 teaspoon cold-pressed sesame seed oil

10 drops sandalwood essential oil

Place the soapwort, gingerroot, and the chamomile flowers in a bowl and cover with the water. Cover the bowl and steep overnight. Strain, discarding the herbal matter. Whip in the sesame oil and sandalwood essential oil. Apply to damp hair. This shampoo will not yield much lather. Rinse with tepid water, then repeat.

MINERAL-RICH RINSE

1 teaspoon thyme leaves

1 teaspoon nasturtium flowers

2 tablespoons burdock root (chopped finely)

4 cups mineral water

Finely chop the thyme leaves and crush the nasturtium flowers. Place the first three ingredients into a saucepan with the water. Bring to a boil and simmer for 10 minutes. Strain and cool. After shampooing, pour the infusion over your hair, leave covered with a towel for 1 hour, then rinse with tepid water. Air-dry.

❧ Sally's Egg Shampoo and Nettle Rinse

Eggs have been used to cleanse hair for generations due to their moisturizing properties. Even today, egg shampoo is regarded as one of the best hair treatments available.

2 fresh eggs

½ cup mineral water (warmed to body temperature)

1 tablespoon fresh aloe gel

2 tablespoons lemon juice

Make sure that the eggs are at room temperature before you begin (take them out of the refrigerator at least 1 hour before preparing the recipe). Place the eggs, water, aloe, and lemon juice in a blender and process on low for 30 seconds. Apply to wet hair, massaging deeply into the roots and scalp. Rinse with warm water. Use twice a week.

NETTLE RINSE

2 cups fresh young nettle leaves and roots (or 4 nettle tea bags)

1 cup water

Dried nettles can be purchased from all good health food stores, either loose or as herbal tea bags.

Place the nettle leaves and roots in a saucepan. Cover with the water and bring to a boil. Simmer for 5 minutes, then remove from the heat and strain. Either eat the herb or discard. (Or immerse the tea bags in 2 cups of hot water and steep for 15 minutes, squeeze out the bags, saving the tea.) Cool the juice/tea, then apply to your clean hair, rubbing it into the scalp and hair roots. Leave in for 1 hour, then rinse with tepid water. Repeat treatment every other day for 1 week.

Calendula Cradle Cap Lotion

This sweet, aromatic lotion is ideal for treating cradle cap, a common scalp condition in infants. It is also good for adults with oily hair.

2 tablespoons plantain seed infusion

4 tablespoons cold-pressed almond oil

4 tablespoons infused calendula oil

10 drops chamomile essential oil

1 tablespoon aloe gel

Place 1 teaspoon of plantain seeds in 1 cup of very hot water. Cover and steep for 45 minutes. Strain and cool. Measure the almond, infused calendula, and chamomile oils into a small bowl and whip together. Add the aloe gel and stir. Pour the mixture into the plantain seed infusion and whip again. If you've made this lotion for a baby, make sure lotion is neither hot nor cold. Massage into the scalp, paying special attention to trouble spots. Comb through, picking off any loosened scales, then leave on overnight. Do not wash the infant's head with any shampoo during the 7 days of treatment. Adults should part the hair in rows and dab the lotion on the scalp with a soft brush or cotton ball. Leave on overnight and shower off in warm water the following morning.

Shelley's Coconut Dry-End Cream

This enriching cream will not mend split ends; the only way to cure them is to snip them off. But it will temporarily seal them, arresting further splitting along the hair shafts. The ingredients are potent tissue regenerators.

3 tablespoons cocoa butter

3 tablespoons coconut oil

2 tablespoons cold-pressed sweet almond oil

15 drops neroli essential oil

Melt the cocoa butter and coconut oil in the top half of a double boiler on a low heat. Remove and cool. Add the almond oil and whip vigorously. Add the neroli oil, and pour into a sterilized glass jar. Seal and label with contents and date. Store in the refrigerator between uses. Bring to room temperature before each application. Rub small amounts of the cream into the dry, split ends after shampooing and conditioning.

✍ *Herb-Mud Shampoo*

An unusual, deeply cleansing shampoo, the formula purifies and soothes the often malnourished follicles and hair shafts. It is restorative, refreshing, and pH-normalizing, leaving the hair soft and smelling like a spring garden at dusk.

4 tablespoons rhassoul mud (powdered)

2 teaspoons of the following herbs:

     Rosemary leaves

     Sage leaves

     Lavender flower buds

     Nettle leaves and root

½ cup mineral water

1 tablespoon apple cider vinegar diluted in ¼ cup of water

Place the rhassoul mud in a bowl, then set aside. Make a combined infusion of the herbs and water, following the instructions on page 36. Steep for 45 minutes. Strain and pour over the mud and whip vigorously. Pour the diluted cider vinegar into another bowl to use as the final rinse. Massage a small amount of the shampoo into your dampened hair, then pile the remaining on top of your head. Cover your head with a plastic shower cap and a warm towel. Allow mixture to penetrate for 15 minutes. Rinse with warm water and use the diluted vinegar as the final rinse.

Hot Olive Oil Restructurer

For generations, women have applied natural oils to their hair as conditioners. This simple recipe is effective for brittle, dry, heat-damaged, permed, or chemically altered hair. If your hair is so unmanageable that getting a comb through leaves you in tears, tame your mass of tangles with this nourishing treatment twice a week. You'll notice a marked improvement after just one application.

> 3 tablespoons cold-pressed olive oil
>
> 1 tablespoon cold-pressed sesame oil
>
> 1 teaspoon evening primrose oil (pierce and squeeze from 3 capsules)
>
> 1 teaspoon gingerroot juice

Place the olive, sesame, and evening primrose oils into a bowl. Rest the bowl in a saucepan half filled with hot water. Stir the oils as they warm through. Add the ginger juice and whip vigorously. Apply warm, using your fingertips to massage it into your hair, beginning at the nape of your neck and working forward. Cover with a plastic shower cap, then a warmed towel, to trap moisture and body heat. Leave on for 20 minutes. Rinse with warm water. Finish off with a brief cold rinse.

✑ Petula's Antidandruff Rinse

Any dandruff sufferer will tell you that using commercial hair products that are meant to tame hair actually make their dandruff worse. This delightful aromatic recipe works with your body's systems to heal itself naturally.

    1 cup very hot water

    2 tablespoons fresh rosemary leaves (chopped and crushed)

    2 teaspoons borax

    5 drops tea tree essential oil

    5 drops lavender essential oil

    2 drops rosemary essential oil

Measure the hot water into a bowl, then add the rosemary leaves and borax. Cover and steep for 2 hours. Strain, then add the essential oils to the liquid. Recipe yields 1–3 treatments, depending on the length and volume of your hair. Between uses, refrigerate leftovers in a squeeze bottle.

After shampooing and conditioning, rinse your hair with clean, tepid water, then the antidandruff rinse, and wrap your hair in a towel for 45 minutes. Rinse off with warm water, then air-dry.

✑ Chamomile and Lemon Shampoo

This is a sweet smelling, kind shampoo with gentle highlighting properties. Do a strand test (follow the instructions on page 164), as chamomile is used to dye wool and yarn yellow.

¼ cup fresh chamomile flowers

2 cups very hot water

2 tablespoons baby shampoo

1 teaspoon fresh lemon juice

2 teaspoons nettle root decoction

Place the chamomile flowers into a bowl and cover with the hot water. Cover and steep for 30 minutes, then strain the infusion into a bowl and discard the flowers. Measure the baby shampoo and lemon juice into a bowl and stir gently. Make the nettle root decoction (follow instructions on page 39), then cool and add the chamomile infusion. Whip vigorously, then add the lemon juice mixture. Massage into damp hair, working from the nape of your neck forward. Leave on for 5 minutes, then rinse with tepid water. Use every other day to maximize highlight effects.

Molasses Intensive Hair Conditioner

Here's another concentrated, unconventional hair treatment for the scalp that works well on dry, brittle, and heat-damaged hair.

3 tablespoons cold-pressed sweet almond oil

3 teaspoons blackstrap molasses

2 egg yolks

2 teaspoons aloe gel

Measure the almond oil, molasses, and egg yolks into a small bowl and whip vigorously. Add the aloe, and stir to form a smooth paste. Apply to dry, clean hair. Part your hair in rows and use an old brush to cover your whole head. Cover your treated hair with a plastic shower cap and a warmed towel to trap moisture and body heat. Leave on for 30 minutes. Rinse with warm water, finishing with a brief, tepid rinse. Air-dry.

Eat a plentiful diet of the following raw vegetables:

Watercress leaves

Broccoli florets

Dandelion leaves

Radish

Beet tops

All sulfur-rich foods bind amino acids in the hair shafts. Eat plenty of raw onions, too, or rub a raw onion on your hair before shampooing.

❧ *Stimulating Hair Growth Conditioner*

Good for all hair types, this delicately scented conditioner can be used daily. The potent essential oils stimulate blood circulation in the scalp and effectively remove dandruff or other scaling skin conditions.

> 4 tablespoons cold-pressed grape seed oil
> 5 drops (each) of the following essential oils:
> > Lemon balm (melissa)
> > Rosemary
> > Lavender
> > Basil
> > Clary sage
> > Ylang ylang
> 4 tablespoons burdock root decoction

Measure the grape seed oil into a bowl and add the essential oils. Gently whisk. Bring the burdock decoction to a boil, then simmer for 30 minutes or until the liquid has reduced by one-third. Strain the liquid into a bowl, then either eat the delicious herb or discard it. Cool the decoction, then add it to the oil mixture and whip gently.

Pour about 1 tablespoon of the mixture into the palm of your hand and massage it into your scalp. Focus on the scalp and hair ends; you need not coat the length of every strand. Cover with a plastic shower cap and leave it on for 30 minutes. Rinse with warm water.

✍ Christine's Dry Shampoo Formulas

For all those times when washing your hair is inconvenient, try these recipes, which give your hair a lustrous shine. All are good hair treatments for busy travelers.

ORRISROOT AND CITRUS GRANULES

1 teaspoon orrisroot (powered)

1 teaspoon lemon zest (finely grated)

Combine the ingredients and store in a small, sterilized, shallow glass jar and place in a warm, dry place for 1 week. Shake jar daily.

Part dry, brushed hair at the center and sprinkle a bit of the shampoo on the hair. Massage with your fingertips, then leave on for 15 minutes. Turn your head upside down and vigorously brush the tiny particles out. Any grime, grease, or dead skin cells are brushed out, too.

LIME AND BASIL SHAMPOO GRANULES

2 tablespoons fresh basil leaves (chopped finely)

Zest of 1 lime (grated finely)

1 teaspoon baking soda

1 teaspoon fine sugar granules

Combine ingredients in a small, sterilized, shallow glass jar. Store for 1 week, then apply as above.

SEMOLINA AND LAVENDER BUD SHAMPOO

1 teaspoon fresh lavender buds

1 tablespoon semolina

½ teaspoon baking soda

Bruise lavender buds by crushing them with the back of a spoon. Combine ingredients in a small, sterilized glass jar. Store for 1 week, then apply as above.

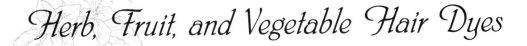

Herb, Fruit, and Vegetable Hair Dyes

*H*air dyes and rinses made with herbal infusions, fruit, vegetables, and natural minerals are beginning to pop up on the shelves in natural food stores. If you haven't seen these products and want to create a custom color, or you're just simply looking for a jolly good time, the following recipes are for you. Some of these preparations are a little complicated to master, and they're all messy fun.

Whichever herbal, fruit, or vegetable dye, highlighter, tint, or combination preparation you plan to use, it is important to do a test on a few strands of hair before taking the plunge and slathering it on. Each person's hair type is different, even people within the same family. Your hair might take on a very different shade than your sister's or child's hair, even when you use the same treatment. Remember to protect countertops and other surfaces where you prepare and apply these recipes. Their aim is to color your hair, not your hands. Discover a whole new world of beautifying possibilities on the following pages.

Guidelines

Protect Yourself Always wear plastic or latex gloves when massaging the natural pastes and rinses into your hair. Cover countertops with newspaper. There are no skin-damaging chemicals in these treatments, but the natural pigments will stain clothing, countertops, and hands.

Perform a Strand Test Always, always perform a strand test before applying a preparation to your whole head. If your skin is sensitive, perform a skin patch test (see page 34), too.

Recycle Use old towels and application brushes. Use a warm towel to cover your treated hair. It helps to keep your body heat and the moisture locked in while the dye takes effect.

Water   When a recipe calls for water as an ingredient, do not use tap water unless it is filtered. Chemicals in untreated water will react with the natural ingredients in the dye mix, sometimes with disastrous results. It's best to use distilled or bottled water. Boil and cool water before use.

Read the Instructions   You'll want to have everything you need handy. Carefully read the instructions before you begin.

❧ Herb and Henna Dyes

Henna can produce a wide range of hair colors, depending on the natural color and chemistry of your own hair and the color potency life force of the henna you use in your recipe. Combining henna with other natural ingredients such as fruit, flowers, leaves, and root pigments expands the range of tints and tones you can produce. By substituting strong teas and coffee for water, you are able to tone down some of the fiery reds and oranges to softer browns and auburn. Some hair types absorb these dyes more quickly than others, but like all natural, living preparations, henna's effects will vary. The climate and soil in which it was grown affect its dyeing properties. Making and using herbal, fruit, and vegetable hair dyes is more labor-intensive than buying commercial coloring mixes, but they're free of harsh chemicals, actually improve hair texture, and are soothing to the scalp.

❧ A Natural World of Colors

Here's a basic recipe to get you started:

   ½ oz. powdered henna leaves

   1 oz. herb or spice dye (see list below)

   1½ cups distilled or bottled water (or strong black coffee/tea)

   2 tablespoons sweet almond oil

Place the powdered henna leaves and other dry ingredients into a saucepan. Boil the water (or strong coffee or tea) and remove from heat. Dissolve the herbs into the solution, a little at a time. Add the almond oil, and give the paste a vigorous mix. Use all the mixture in one application. Part your clean, damp hair into sections and apply the color with a soft brush. Start at the roots, but cover the length of each strand. Place a plastic cap over your pasted hair and secure it. Cover the cap with a warm towel. Leave the dye on your hair for 35 minutes. The longer the dye remains on your hair, the darker and more prominent the color will be. Rinse with warm water, until the water runs clear. More than one application may be necessary to achieve the color, shade, or tint you desire.

Natural Plant Hair Dyes   These earth-wise plant-origin dyes work with your natural hair chemistry to produce subtle or daring shades and colors. They contain no harsh chemical bleaching agents. Therefore, if your natural hair color is black or dark brown, applying a gentle lightening paste of chamomile, rhubarb, or safflower will have little effect. On the other hand, you can achieve striking effects by applying one of the reddening or darkening pastes to blond or light brown hair colors.

Herb, Spice, Fruit, and Vegetable Dying Pigments

PLANT SOURCE	PART USED	COLOR ACHIEVED	ADVICE
Alkanet	root	red brown	Good for all hair types
Annanot	seeds	red	Will cover blonds and tint dark hair
Artichoke	leaves	brown	Will cover light hair and tint dark types
Chamomile	flowers	honey blond	Not appropriate for black/dark brown hair
Gallnut	gall	brown	Will shade dark hair and color light hair
Henna	leaves	copper	Will cover light hair and tint black hair

Indigo	leaves	blue black	Not appropriate for blond hair
Ivy	leaves	brown	Will shade dark hair and cover light hair
Logwood	wood	copper	Not appropriate for light blond hair
Madder	root	bright red	Not appropriate for light blond hair
Quebracho	bark/wood	deep red	Will cover light hair and tint darker hair
Rhubarb	root and stem	golden blond	Not appropriate for black or brown hair
Safflower	flowers	orange yellow	Will not tint or shade black or brown hair
Turmeric	root	yellow blond	Not for dark hair types
Walnut	leaves	brown	Will color and shade all hair colors
Walnut husks	husks	brown	Will shade dark hair and color light hair

❧ Natural Dye Allergy Test

Skin allergies can develop quite unexpectedly. This test must therefore be performed at least forty-eight hours before applying a natural herbal dye. You will need a cotton swab or cotton ball, small saucer or bowl, and a spoon. Make up a quarter of the coloring recipe that you intend to use on your hair. Dab the cotton swab or ball into the coloring mixture, then apply to a soft patch of skin on your arm. Hold in place for two to three minutes, then remove. Leave the area of skin uncovered for at least forty-eight hours. If an itchy rash, burning sensation, or redness occurs, you may be allergic to one or more of the natural ingredients in the recipe, and you must not use this preparation on your scalp. Cover the sore area of skin with a calendula and comfrey infusion, then leave it to air-dry. Use the remaining dye for the following hair strand test.

ᕺ *Hair Strand Test*

You need to perform this simple test on a clipping of your hair to find out how long to leave the color paste or rinse on your hair to achieve the result you want. Do this test every time you color your hair. You will need a small pair of scissors, some tape, and one plastic glove. Cut a quarter-inch-wide strand of clean, dry hair from the grayest or darkest area of your hair, close to the scalp. Place the tape over the cut end, then put on the plastic glove. With the remaining mixture from the allergy test, dip the hair strand into the mixture so it's completely covered. Start timing. After fifteen minutes, wipe the hair strand clean. If it is not the color or shade you want, return it to the mixture and check its progress every three minutes, up to a maximum of forty-five minutes. If the color is too fiery, you can add coffee or tea to tone it down. Hard-to-color areas of gray hair may need longer coloring time than other parts. When you have achieved the color you want, make a note of the time it took so that you can repeat the duration with your whole head.

ᕺ *Pamela's Hibiscus Rinse*

For all brown and auburn hair colors and types, use this simple rinse for reddish highlights.

3 cups water

4 tablespoons dried hibiscus flowers

Boil the water, remove from the heat, and cool for 5 minutes before immersing the hibiscus flowers. Cover and steep for 25 minutes. Place over a low heat and simmer for 15 minutes. Remove from the heat, cover, and further steep for 45 minutes. Massage into hair with your hands, then cover with a shower cap and warmed towel. Relax for 20 minutes or more, depending on the shade you want to achieve. Rinse thoroughly with warm water, until the water runs clear.

Brunettes can drink the following herbal infusion twice a day to restore natural pH and nourish the follicles.

    1 cup of water
    2 teaspoons unhulled sesame seeds
    ¼ cup burdock root (chopped)

Measure the water into a small saucepan and add the sesame seeds and chopped burdock root. Bring to a boil, reduce the heat, and simmer for 20 minutes. Remove from the heat and cool before drinking.

Rosemary-Walnut Blackening Paste

For mature heads of graying dark brown and black hair, this natural dye is for you. Remove telltale signs of aging with the twice-monthly application of this paste. Both red sage and green walnut skins can be purchased dried through mail order suppliers.

    1 cup green walnut skins
    6 tablespoons brandy
    1 teaspoon red sage
    6 drops rosemary essential oil

If using fresh walnut skins, chop them finely, then crush them, using the back of a wooden spoon or pestle. For dried skins, hydrate them in ½ cup of warm water for 10 minutes, drain, then chop finely and crush. Mix with the brandy and pour into a sterilized bottle. Seal and label with contents and date. Leave to macerate for 2 weeks, shaking the jar daily. Make an infusion of the red sage following the instructions on page 36. Cover and steep for 30 minutes, strain, then set aside. Empty the jar of macerated walnut skins into a bowl, then add the rosemary essential oil. Now add the sage infusion. Whip lightly with a whisk.

Using a clean makeup brush or flat paintbrush, apply the paste, beginning at the roots and working out to the ends. Pay special attention to graying areas. Cover your hair with a plastic shower cap, then a towel, to trap body heat and moisture. Relax for 30 minutes. Rinse with warm water until it runs clear.

✑ Reddening Paste and Nasturtium Rinse

This potent coloring paste will enhance golden and fiery red hair and highlight your natural hair color, whatever it may be.

½ cup Iranian henna (powdered)

2 tablespoons ground coffee

1 cup very hot water

1 egg yolk

1 tablespoon strong sage leaf infusion (see instructions on page 36)

2 teaspoons cold-pressed sweet almond oil

In a bowl, mix the henna with the coffee. Add enough hot water to make a smooth paste. Add the lightly beaten egg and sage infusion, then beat again.

Massage clean, dry hair with the almond oil to prevent drying. Using a small, flat brush, apply the paste, starting at the roots and working your way through to the ends. Put on a plastic shower cap, then cover your head with a warm towel. Leave on for 45 minutes, less time to achieve a lighter shade, more time for a darker tone. Rinse with warm water, until it runs clear.

½ cup nasturtium flower and leaf infusion

½ cup nettle leaf and root infusion

Allow each infusion to steep, covered, for 30 minutes. Strain through a fine mesh into a single pitcher. Pour over hair, leave in for 15 minutes, then rinse with tepid water.

❧ *Olive's Lightening Paste and Mullein Rinse*

This clay-based paste for blonds and light brown hair will lighten fair shades. You may need two or three applications to achieve the desired color. Chamomile has been used for centuries to dye yarn and fiber, and many women use a fresh chamomile infusion before or after shampooing to highlight their naturally light-colored hair.

½ cup fresh chamomile flowers

1 cup very hot water (for infusion)

4 sticks rhubarb with white root tops (boiled, then simmered for 15 minutes, and cooled)

1 egg yolk

1 cup kaolin clay

Place the chamomile flowers in a bowl, then pour over the hot water. Cover and steep for 30 minutes. Cook, strain, and mash the rhubarb. Beat the egg yolk. Strain the chamomile infusion. Combine the egg, chamomile, rhubarb, and kaolin clay in a bowl, then whip into a smooth paste. Set aside, covered. On dry hair, apply the paste, using a flat brush and working from the roots to the ends. Cover with a plastic shower cap, then a towel, and let it penetrate for 30–45 minutes. Rinse with warm water until it runs clear.

¼ cup mullein flower infusion

½ cup marigold flower infusion

1 tablespoon fresh lemon juice

Cover and steep the combined flower infusion (see instructions for making flower infusions on page 36) for 30 minutes. Strain, then mix with the lemon juice. Apply as a final rinse after the coloring paste. Leave on hair for 15 minutes, then rinse with tepid water.

✍ Ed's Tobacco Rinse and Color-Restoring Tea

This simple herbal (yes, tobacco is an herb) rinse for graying hair encourages your natural color to shine through. It's especially effective on auburn or brown hair.

½ cup Darjeeling tea

2 tablespoons loose, dry, dark tobacco (not chewing tobacco)

2 cups very hot water

Make the tea by immersing 5 tea bags into 2 cups of very hot water. Leave to steep for 30 minutes. Place the loose tobacco into the 2 cups of hot water and leave covered for 15 minutes. (If you are attempting to cover all your gray hair, allow the tobacco to steep for 30–45 minutes.) Strain the Darjeeling tea and the tobacco infusion, then combine.

Pour the tobacco rinse over clean, wet hair and massage it in with your fingertips. Cover your hair with a plastic shower cap, then a towel, and leave them on for 15 minutes. Rinse with tepid water, then blot excess with an old towel. Air-dry.

2 tablespoons dandelion leaf infusion

2 tablespoons horsetail infusion

2 tablespoons nettle leaf infusion

Drink an 8-oz. glass of this cell-regenerating infusion twice a day. All of these hedgerow herbs are abundantly rich in silica and skin-nutritious beta-carotene.

Barbara's Orange-Walnut Paste and Safflower Coloring Rinse

For all dark blond and light brown hair types, use this sweet-smelling paste in early fall, when walnuts are abundant. You may need two or three applications to achieve the desired shade.

5 tablespoons chopped green walnut skins

3 tablespoons alum crystals (powdered)

1 tablespoon aloe gel

½ cup orange flower water

1 egg yolk (lightly beaten)

Bruise the fresh walnut skins, then chop finely and transfer to a bowl. Soak dried walnut skins in ½ cup of very hot water for 5 minutes. Strain, then chop finely. Sprinkle the powdered alum crystals over the walnut skins, add the aloe, then pour in the orange flower water. Stir, then add the egg and beat into a smooth paste.

Part clean, damp hair, then, using a soft brush to apply the paste, begin at the roots and work through to the ends. Cover with a plastic shower cap, then a warm towel and relax for 45 minutes. Rinse with tepid water, until it runs clear. Towel dry.

HERBAL CONDITIONING INFUSION

4 tablespoons safflower infusion

4 tablespoons rhubarb stalk infusion

Make a combined infusion of the herbs. Cover and steep for 30 minutes. Strain and pour over your colored hair. Massage into the scalp for 10 minutes. Comb through, then rinse with tepid water. Air-dry.

ᔕ *Victoria's Mullein Paste and Chamomile Final Rinse*

This deeply cleansing paste for dark blond and light brown hair brings out golden tints and highlights beautifully.

1 ½ cups strong Darjeeling tea

2 tablespoons mullein leaves (dried and powdered)

2 tablespoons fuller's earth

1 teaspoon aloe gel

1 teaspoon cold-pressed sweet almond oil

Make the Darjeeling tea by immersing 5 tea bags in 2 cups of very hot water. Steep for 15 minutes, then strain. Place the infusion in a small saucepan, then sprinkle in the mullein herb. Simmer for 20 minutes, then remove from heat. Once cooled, strain into a bowl and add the fuller's earth and aloe gel. Beat into a smooth paste.

Cover your hands with the almond oil and massage it through your hair. Comb your hair, then part it in rows and apply the paste with a soft brush, working from the roots to the ends. Cover your hair and relax for 45 minutes (depending on the shade you wish to achieve). Rinse with tepid water and towel off excess.

Beautiful Face, Beautiful Body

FINAL RINSE

4 tablespoons chamomile flower infusion

4 tablespoons safflower infusion

Cover and steep for 30 minutes, then strain. Pour over your hair as a final, color-enhancing rinse. Leave on for 15 minutes, then wash out with tepid water. Air-dry.

Rhubarb Highlight Paste and Geranium Color-Enhancing Rinse

This scalp-soothing paste for light brown and golden blond hair lightens and conditions. It is recommended for fair-hair types as the rhubarb has remarkable natural bleaching properties. If your hair color is light brown or dark blond, you may need three or four applications to achieve a glistening highlight effect.

1 large rhubarb stick and root

3 tablespoons kaolin clay

2 teaspoons glycerin

2 cups water

1 egg yolk

1 teaspoon cider vinegar

Chop the rhubarb finely, then crush it with the back of a wooden spoon. Place the kaolin in a small bowl, then add the glycerin and stir. Pour the water into a small saucepan with the rhubarb and simmer for 25 minutes. Strain through a fine mesh (either eat the fruit or discard it). Beat the egg yolk, then add it to the kaolin mix. Once rhubarb infusion has cooled, add to the paste with the cider vinegar. Whip gently with a hand whisk. Apply the paste to clean, dry hair, parting it from the crown forward. Spread paste through from the roots to the ends, then cover your hair and leave it for 45 minutes. Rinse with warm water.

FINAL RINSE

½ cup geranium infusion

Allow infusion to steep, covered, for 30 minutes. Strain, then pour over hair and leave in.

❧ Henna-Indigo Paste and Sage Rinse

This thick, darkening paste for gray and dark brown hair will blacken your hair and give off reddish brown specks as the henna highlights. It produces a lustrous shine and silky texture.

2 cups very hot water

12 tablespoons red henna powder

1 cup indigo leaves (powdered)

1 egg yolk, lightly beaten

1 teaspoon fuller's earth (if mixture is too runny)

2 teaspoons cold-pressed jojoba bean oil (to massage into scalp to prevent drying)

Measure the water into a bowl, then add the henna and powdered indigo. Cover and steep for 15 minutes. Lightly beat the egg yolk and set aside. Once the herb infusion is cool, add the egg and beat into a smooth paste. If the paste is too runny, sprinkle 1 teaspoon of fuller's earth into the mixture.

Massage your scalp and hair ends with the jojoba bean oil before applying the paste. Part your hair in sections and, using a soft, flat brush, cover your hair from the roots to the ends. Relax for 45 minutes to 1 hour. Rinse with warm water and towel off excess.

FINAL RINSE

½ cup red sage infusion

Pour cooled infusion over your hair, massage through gently, then leave in for 15 minutes before rinsing with tepid water. Blot with an old towel, then air-dry.

Chamomile Lightening Paste and Prepaste Color Stay Infusion

This delicate, sweet-smelling highlighter for blond and light brown hair soothes the scalp and regenerates hair follicles. It gives hair an irresistible sheen and healthy luster.

PREPASTE INFUSION

4 tablespoons lavender flower infusion

4 tablespoons mullein flower infusion

4 tablespoons safflower infusion

Make a combined infusion. Cover and steep for 30 minutes.

1 cup fresh chamomile flowers

2 cups very hot water

10 tablespoons kaolin clay

1 egg yolk

1 tablespoon aloe gel

2 tablespoons marigold flower infusion (see instructions on page 36)

2 teaspoons cold-pressed sunflower seed oil

Place the fresh (or dried) chamomile flowers into a saucepan, then pour the very hot water over them. Cover and steep for 5 minutes. Simmer over a low heat for 15 minutes. Strain and then let it stand for 15 minutes. Sprinkle the kaolin clay over the chamomile infusion in a bowl and mix. Beat together the egg yolk, aloe, and marigold infusion, then add to the kaolin mixture and whip vigorously.

Now you're ready to begin the treatment. Strain the infusion and pour over dry hair. Massage into hair and scalp. Leave for 10 minutes. Now massage in the sunflower oil into hair and scalp using your fingertips. Apply the paste, using a small, flat brush. Start at the roots and work through to the ends. Once covered, trap the moisture and body heat with a plastic shower cap and warm towel. Leave hair covered so paste can penetrate for 45 minutes. Rinse with warm water until it runs clear, and towel off excess. Air-dry.

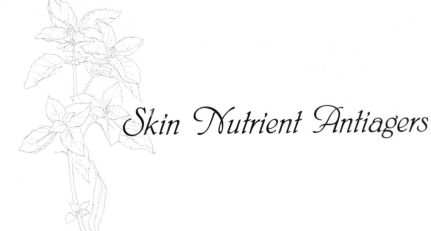

Skin Nutrient Antiagers

*Y*our skin is a living, breathing suit. Facials, masks, body wraps, toners, astringents, and exfoliants treat more than just the skin's surface. Their active ingredients penetrate and are absorbed into the outer and deeper dermal layers and bloodstream. Much of what you apply to your skin works its way through your whole body. Likewise, whatever you feed your body shows up in the condition and texture of your skin. So treat your skin right! Feed it with good food and enrich your skin with micronutrient-packed facials, creams, rejuvenating compresses, and sunblocks that counteract photo-aging and skin malnutrition.

Photo-aging describes what happens to human skin prematurely aged by the sun. Overexposure to the sun is preventable. Cover up and save your ageless skin. Why let the sun turn your beautiful face and body into a dry, malnourished, wrinkled mess? The sun damages the skin from the outside in, reducing the distribution, production, and quantity of oil secretions, thinning the dermis and disrupting the healthy production of immune cells that fight infection. Photo-aged skin becomes vulnerable to disease and accelerated degeneration.

To keep your ageless, beautiful skin all your life, follow these simple rules.

1. Drink lots of water to provide the moisture needed to plump up your skin.
2. Hydrate your skin from the outside with moisture-attracting ingredients such as aloe and honey in the form of facials and cleansers.
3. Seal in skin moisture with oils that contain essential fatty acids. Jojoba bean oil (which is both waxy and oily) is the best, as it is very similar to the skin's natural sebum.
4. Get at least six to eight hours of sleep every night.
5. Exfoliate. For ageless skin, you should exfoliate more than once a day. Try brushing dry skin before cleansing. Exfoliate as you cleanse with an exfoliating cleanser, loofah, or sea sponge. You can't do it too much.
6. Eat lots of raw vegetables and fruit.

7. Don't smoke. Smoking destroys vitamin C, which keeps collagen fibers strong and healthy.
8. Wear a sunscreen (SPF 15) daily.

ᔕ *Chamomile Eye Tonic*

This is the perfect tonic for puffy, tired eyes. Chamomile nourishes skin and regenerates cells, and the witch hazel is soothing. This tonic will leave the delicate tissues surrounding the lashes and brows feeling silky smooth.

2 tablespoons chamomile flower infusion (see instructions on page 36)

1 teaspoon cold-pressed castor oil

1 teaspoon fresh aloe gel

5 drops frankincense essential oil

2 drops chamomile essential oil

1 tablespoon distilled witch hazel

Cover and steep the chamomile infusion for 30 minutes, then strain. Save the chamomile flowers and put them in a piece of muslin or cotton gauze and place them in the refrigerator for 5 minutes. Place the castor oil and aloe gel into a saucer and mash. Transfer into a bowl and add the frankincense and chamomile essential oils; whisk gently. Before applying the eye tonic, place the cooled poultice over closed lids and rest for 15 minutes. Remove the poultice and air-dry.

Using the tips of your index fingers, dab small amounts of the Chamomile Eye Tonic over the delicate skin, working from the outside in on the lower eye tissue, and from the inside out on the upper eye tissue. I like to follow with a generous treatment of the Cornflower Mist (page 69).

✒ Carrot Wrinkle Soother

This is a potent, sensual, and soothing night cream for those creases otherwise known as squints and laughter lines.

½ teaspoon of the following oils:

    Avocado (cold-pressed)

    Carrot (macerated)

    Castor (cold-pressed)

    Evening primrose (infused)

    Marigold (infused)

    Saint-John's-wort (infused)

    Wheat germ (cold-pressed)

1 teaspoon beeswax pearls

1 teaspoon lavender blossom honey

1 teaspoon shea butter

1 teaspoon cocoa butter

Measure all the ingredients into the top half of a double boiler and heat through, stirring occasionally. Remove from the heat when the beeswax, cocoa butter, and shea butter have completely melted. Whisk to form a smooth paste.

Massage the carrot cream into creases around your mouth, eyes, nose, and chin with your fingertips. Start off with the Fennel Eye Bath (page 69) for a super anti-wrinkle treatment.

Beautiful Face, Beautiful Body

❧ Molly's Quick-Fix Facial

This recipe will give your whole face an instant moisture fix. I like to start with the Herb Milk Mist (page 70).

1 small avocado (very ripe)
1 teaspoon cold-pressed olive oil
1 egg yolk
2 teaspoons aloe gel

Cut the avocado in half and remove the stone. Scoop out the soft flesh with a small spoon and place it into a bowl. Add the olive oil, egg yolk, and aloe. Beat vigorously into a smooth paste. Apply the paste with a small, flat brush or your fingertips. Exfoliate with the avocado skin and stone by rubbing them over your pasted face for a few minutes.

Apply the paste with your fingers. Air-dry for 15 minutes, then rinse with warm water and pat dry.

❧ Reggie's Raw Potato Eye Compress

Eyes depend on good circulation to keep them twinkling and supplied with the nutrients they need. Herbal infusions, baths, washes, and teas also help to refresh and soothe your eyes, toning the tiny muscles. This simple, living recipe will soothe, heal, and refresh, keeping your windows to the soul bright and healthy.

4 small new potatoes

½ cup strong chamomile infusion (see instructions on page 36)

¼ cup fresh aloe gel

Grate the potatoes into a bowl, then stir in the chamomile infusion and aloe gel. Toss a muslin cloth or sterilized cotton gauze into the mixture and refrigerate for 10 minutes.

Remove the muslin cloth or gauze from the mixture and rub it over your face. Rinse the cloth and dampen it again in the mixture. Rest the cloth over your eyes and relax for 15 minutes. Rinse with warm water and pat dry.

DIETARY HELP

¼ cup fresh carrot juice

¼ cup fresh bilberry juice

Drink 2 small glasses daily to keep your vision sharp. Carrots and bilberries are considered super foods for the eyes.

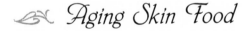 *Aging Skin Food*

This aromatic, skin-nourishing cream is full of concentrated foods the skin craves. Together, they work to repair and regenerate while you sleep.

2 tablespoons cocoa butter

2 tablespoons lanolin

3 teaspoons cold-pressed avocado oil

3 teaspoons cold-pressed wheat germ oil

4 evening primrose oil capsules

5 drops frankincense essential oil

5 drops neroli essential oil

Measure the cocoa butter and lanolin into the top half of a double boiler. Heat over a low flame. Once melted, remove from the heat and whisk in the avocado and wheat germ oils. Pierce and squeeze the contents of the evening primrose oil capsules into the mixture. Once cool, add the essential oils and whip again.

Moisten skin (try the Fruit Juice Mist on page 70), then gently massage cream into your skin, until completely absorbed. Do not rub your face with any pressure, just lightly glide your finger over its surface in circular motions. Leave on overnight.

ᴁ *Aaron's Youth-Dew Beauty Fluid*

This is one of my favorite recipes. You can triple the ingredients and make enough for a whole week of skin pampering. Store in a glass bottle in the refrigerator between uses.

2 half-inch-thick slices of rye bread (crusts removed)

2 cups apple cider vinegar

2 egg whites

20 drops benzoin tincture

Tear the bread into chunks and place in a bowl with the vinegar. Cover and leave for 10 minutes. Lightly beat the egg whites, then place them in a blender with the soaked bread and vinegar. Process on a low speed for 30 seconds. Strain through a fine mesh, then funnel into a glass bottle. Drop the benzoin tincture into the solution and shake well. Run a warm bath, pour ½ cup of the beauty fluid into the water, then immerse yourself and luxuriate. After bathing, splash your skin with the remaining. Blot excess and air-dry.

❧ Citrus Skin Revitalizer

This tropically scented recipe stimulates pressure points on the face and boosts lymphatic drainage and blood circulation.

    1 small, ripe avocado

    1 teaspoon orange flower honey

    3 teaspoons live-culture yogurt

    3 teaspoons fresh aloe gel

    1 teaspoon fresh lemon juice

Halve the avocado and remove the stone. Scoop the flesh into a bowl and mash. Save skin and stone. Add honey to the mashed fruit, then add the yogurt and aloe. Beat gently to form a smooth paste. Add the lemon juice a little at a time, and beat again. Place the avocado skin and stone in the refrigerator for 10 minutes. Smooth the paste over your whole face, leaving bare-skin circles around your eyes and mouth. Using the chilled avocado stone and skin, begin alternating to exfoliate and soothe your face with gentle rubs and massage, dislodging dead skin cells. Leave for 10 minutes, then rinse with warm water. Splash your face with tepid water, then pat dry.

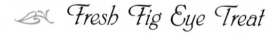 Fresh Fig Eye Treat

This is a simple, utterly delicious, and refreshing treat for tired eyes.

    1 fresh fig (halved)

While your skin is moist (try the Comfrey-Apricot Mist, page 70 to start), place the fig halves over each eye and relax for 15–20 minutes. Rinse with cool water and pat dry.

Beautiful Face, Beautiful Body

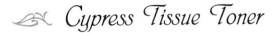 *Cypress Tissue Toner*

This recipe uses a warm poultice to draw excess fluid from puffy eyes. Its firms up slackened skin and reduces wrinkles.

4 tablespoons cracked linseeds

¼ cup very hot water

5 drops cypress essential oil

Fine muslin or sterilized cotton gauze

2 slices of fresh cucumber

Crack open and grind the linseeds in a coffee grinder or ice crusher, then transfer to a bowl. Cover with hot water. Cover and steep for 20 minutes, stirring occasionally as a thick gel begins to form. Once the mixture is cool, add the cypress essential oil and stir. Spoon the aromatic mixture onto muslin or cotton gauze. Place two slices of fresh cucumber over each eye, then carefully lift the edges of the cloth and place the poultice over your face (cloth side down). Place a small warmed towel over your whole face and relax for 15 minutes. Remove poultice and cucumber and mist your face with tepid water. Pat dry.

Vitamin E-Comfrey Compress and Sore Eye Wash

Try this simple, refreshing herbal treat.

½ cup comfrey leaf infusion (made with 2 tea bags)

1 tablespoon cornflower infusion

2 tablespoons sesame seed infusion

1 teaspoon honey

3 teaspoons cold-pressed wheat germ oil

Steep 2 comfrey tea bags in ½ cup of hot water for 15 minutes. Make the corn-flower and sesame seed infusions by following the instructions on page 36. Cover and steep for 15 minutes, then funnel into a spray bottle and refrigerate for 10 minutes. Add honey to the comfrey infusion. Place the comfrey tea bags into the comfrey-honey solu-tion to soak. Remove the herbal mist from the refrigerator and cover your eyes and face with it. Air-dry for a few minutes, then dab a little wheat germ oil over your lips and the tissue surrounding your eyes. Place the soaked comfrey tea bags over each eye and relax for 10 minutes.

SORE EYE WASH

4 tablespoons cornflower infusion

4 tablespoons plantain leaf infusion

1 tablespoon eyebright infusion

1 tablespoon chamomile infusion

After steeping each infusion for 30 minutes, combine and strain through a fine mesh. Pour it into a bowl and refrigerate. Soak a muslin cloth or cotton diaper in the solution. Cover your eyes with the cloth and leave for 5 minutes. Rinse cloth and repeat.

Beautiful Face, Beautiful Body

Witch Hazel Skin Firmer

First used by Elizabethan women, this recipe has grown more popular with each successive generation. Left on the facial skin all day, it gives your complexion a glossy, smooth appearance.

1 teaspoon cider vinegar

3 tablespoons distilled witch hazel

1 egg white

Mix the vinegar and the witch hazel together in a bowl, then lightly beat in the egg whites. Whip until foamy. Refrigerate for 5 minutes. Apply to warm, moist skin with a cotton ball, then leave to air-dry.

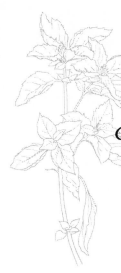

Problem Skin Remedies

*B*eautiful skin draws its sustenance from the foods you eat. Herbal teas, raw fruits and vegetables, and other natural foods provide the nutritional building blocks for soft, clear skin. For the problems that arise from poor hygiene, bad diet, and stress, I offer the following remedies. Soothing, moisturizing, and healing, they work with the body at a cellular level to regenerate and reconstruct with the nutrients it needs most.

Aging is a slow process. The better care you take of your body, the slower the process. Eat well, exercise, relax, drink lots of water, and supplement with vitamins, minerals, enzymes, and needed proteins, and you'll look and feel young for a very long time. When things go wrong, there is always nature to turn to for answers. Recipes and remedies rich in antiseptic botanicals reduce dryness, counteract photo-aging, and prevent collagen depletion. Whatever the skin disorder, there is a healing agent in nature's pharmacy.

✐ Tom's Inside-Out Acne Tonic

Herbalists have long used herbal decoctions for the treatment of acne. No one knows for sure what causes acne, but there is a link between excessive oil secretion, stress, diet, and hormone production. During puberty, high hormone levels trigger a chain reaction, stimulating the sebaceous glands to produce more oil. The following recipe will clear up any persistent acne after 7–10 days.

3 tablespoons of the following herbs:
>   Blue flag
>
>   Cleavers
>
>   Echinacea flowers
>
>   Figwort

2 cups very hot water

3 teaspoons fresh aloe juice

Combine the first four ingredients. Measure 3 tablespoons of the mixture into a bowl and store the excess in a dark-colored glass bottle. Cover the herbs with the hot water. Cover and steep for 30 minutes. Strain and discard the herb matter. Add the aloe juice and whisk. Drink the infusion three times a day, twenty minutes after each meal, for ten days.

EXTERNAL ACNE TREATMENTS

Dab the affected areas with one of the following undiluted remedies and leave for 5 minutes, then rinse with tepid water and pat dry.

Fresh lemon juice (to cleanse and detoxify), three times a day

Fresh garlic juice (to dry any weeping spots), twice daily (garlic is a natural antibiotic)

Freshly beaten egg yolk (to nourish and dry), twice a day

Ice water (to cleanse and shrink); mist acne lesions twice daily

Propolis Chapped Lip Salve

This is a wonderful, healing salve for persistent cold sores and chapped lips. Cocoa butter and shea butter are natural moisturizers, locking water to the skin's surface. The propolis is a powerful anti-inflammatory agent.

- 3 teaspoons beeswax pearls
- 3 teaspoons cocoa butter
- 3 teaspoons shea butter
- 1 teaspoon propolis (powdered)
- 1 teaspoon cold-pressed olive oil
- 2 teaspoons cold-pressed wheat germ oil
- Small lip balm molds

Heat all 6 ingredients in the top half of a double boiler and stir occasionally. Only small amounts of the propolis will actually amalgamate with the other ingredients: most of it will turn a creamy consistency and stay in the bottom. Remove from the heat. You need about 5 small lip balm molds (or plastic syringes with the spout cut off, 10 ml or 15 ml capacity works well). Remember to grease the molds with a little oil before pouring in the mixture. Once cool, but not hard, pour the mixture into the molds, then place in the freezer to harden. You can add a few drops of natural flavors, such as lemon and orange, or colors, such as carrot and beet root, but these ingredients are optional. Personally, I like this salve unscented and uncolored.

⨋ Calendula Eczema Oil and Itchy Lesion Bath

Eczema or dry, scaly, and itchy skin, affects millions. There is a link between food sensitivities, such as dairy and wheat. If your eczema flares up occasionally, it might be worthwhile to keep a food log to see if the problem's diet-related. Stress and the deficiency of essential fatty acids are other common causes. This all-ages remedy relieves itching and scaling and soothes the skin's surface.

- 1 teaspoon chickweed infused oil
- 1 teaspoon evening primrose oil
- 3 teaspoons Saint-John's-wort infused oil
- 3 teaspoons calendula macerated oil (see page 38 for instructions to make macerated oil)
- 1 teaspoon wheat germ oil

Funnel the oils together into a small, sterilized bottle. Shake before each use.

ITCHY LESION BATH
- 4 tablespoons red clover infusion
- 4 tablespoons burdock root decoction
- 4 tablespoons chickweed infusion
- 2 tablespoons heartease infusion
- 2 tablespoons chamomile (*Matricaria recutita*) infusion
- 2 tablespoons marigold infusion

Make the infusions (see page 36) and decoction (see page 39). Combine the infusions and decoction in a bowl and whisk. Run a hot bath, then pour in the herbal remedy. Soak for 20 minutes. Apply the Calendula Eczema Oil to warm, dry skin.

✑ Witch Hazel Pore Tightener

*T*his bewitching skin tightener reduces the appearance of puffy, open pores, unclogs the skin, and absorbs excess oil.

    2 tablespoons fuller's earth
    2 teaspoons witch hazel
    1 egg white
    3 teaspoons fresh aloe gel

Mist your face with an herbal infusion, such as the Dandelion Flower Mist (page 66) and air-dry. Apply the paste to dry skin. Let the paste harden for 15 minutes. Rinse with warm water and pat dry.

✑ Patsy's Spot Eliminator Formula and Hormone-Balancing Tea

*T*his formula is an excellent treatment for stubborn pimples, especially those lurking around the chin, forehead, and nose. Both blackheads and whiteheads erupt as a sign of cellular discontent. This simple recipe refreshes the skin's surface and reduces the superficial inflammation and allows it to heal and regenerate.

    2 teaspoons garlic macerated oil
    1 teaspoon cold-pressed hazelnut oil
    3 drops peppermint essential oil
    3 drops tea tree essential oil

Measure the oils into a bowl, adding the essential oils last. Scrub your hands and nails with hot water and rinse with cold. Soak a clean washcloth in a bowl of hot water. Wring, then apply the cloth to your face to soften the pimples and dislodge the dirt. As soon as the cloths begins to feel cool, repeat. Now dab the oil on your skin with your fingertips and massage it into your face with small, circular, upward motions. Leave on. Repeat daily until pimples have diminished.

HERBAL HORMONE-BALANCING TEA

1 teaspoon of the following combination in 1 cup hot water:

> Chickweed
>
> Goldenseal
>
> Echinacea root
>
> Periwinkle
>
> Sarsaparilla
>
> Red raspberry leaf
>
> Gingerroot
>
> Palmetto berries
>
> Ginseng root
>
> Capsicum
>
> Licorice root

Drink 1 cup warm herbal infusion twice daily for 7 days.

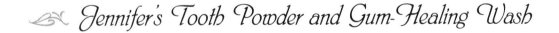

Jennifer's Tooth Powder and Gum-Healing Wash

This dental cleanser formula soothes teeth, gums, and the mouth's soft lining.

> 1 tablespoon orrisroot
>
> 1 tablespoon marshmallow leaves (powdered)
>
> 2 teaspoons dried linden flowers

1 tablespoon freshly ground cinnamon bark

2 tablespoons air-float clay

½ teaspoon propolis

6 drops echinacea tincture

Place the first four ingredients into a blender or food processor (or use a mortar and pestle) to grind into a fine powder. Pass the mixture through a fine-mesh strainer several times to remove any large pieces of plant matter. Add the air-float clay and propolis and stir. Add the echinacea tincture, one drop at a time. Transfer into a small, shallow glass jar and seal. Tip a small amount of the powder into your hand, then dip a moist toothbrush into the powder and brush your teeth and gums thoroughly. Rinse with tepid water.

GUM-HEALING WASH

6 drops myrrh tincture

1 teaspoon prickly ash (powdered)

1 teaspoon bayberry bark (powdered)

4 tablespoons blackberry leaf infusion (see page 36)

Combine the ingredients and pour into a glass bottle. Shake well before use. Pour 1 tablespoon in ½ cup of water and swish around the mouth several times. Do not swallow.

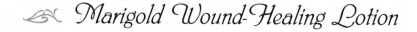

Marigold Wound-Healing Lotion

For cleansing cuts and scrapes on sensitive skin, use this lotion.

2 teaspoons of the following herbs:

    Goldenseal (powdered)

    Garlic (powdered)

    Marigold petals (fresh)

    Pulsatilla

½ cup water

3 drops of the following essential oils:

    Calendula

    Lavender

    Tea tree

Measure the first four ingredients into a small saucepan, then cover with the water. Warm over a low heat and simmer for 15 minutes. Cool, then add the essential oils. Transfer into a small bowl. Dab the affected skin with a cotton ball dipped in the lotion, then air-dry. Any leftovers can be stored in a small jar at room temperature. Discard after 7 days.

Inside-Out Psoriasis Tonic and Plantain Skin Wash

Medical herbalists often cure psoriasis with herbal decoctions and infusions taken daily. Use the wash twice daily and take the tonic three times a day, and you will notice a marked improvement in the appearance and size of those itchy lesions within a few days.

    2 cups very hot water

    3 tablespoons of the following herbs:

        Burdock root

        Chickweed leaves

        Dandelion leaves

        Red clover flowers

        Sarsaparilla flowers

        Yellow dock root

    3 tablespoons fresh aloe juice

Measure the water into a small saucepan, then immerse the herbs and simmer over a low heat for 15 minutes. Strain through a fine mesh, discarding the herb matter, and add the aloe juice. Refrigerate for 5 minutes before drinking. Drink ½ cup of the tonic three times a day before meals.

SKIN WASH

¼ cup plantain leaf infusion

¼ cup nettle leaf infusion

See instructions for making leaf infusions on page 36. Combine infusions, strain, and funnel into a spray bottle. Use immediately in one application and splash over affected skin. Leave to air-dry.

Plant Hormone Healing Lotion

This is another useful treatment for acne-prone complexions.

1 teaspoon cold-pressed avocado oil

1 teaspoon cold-pressed hazelnut oil

1 tablespoon marigold macerated oil (see page 38 for instructions)

1 tablespoon chickweed infused oil

1 teaspoon aloe gel

3 drops tea tree essential oil

3 drops peppermint essential oil

Measure all the ingredients into a bowl and whisk gently. Using a cotton ball soaked in the oil, dab over the affected area. Do not wash off. Use twice daily, morning and night.

Beautiful Face, Beautiful Body

Molly's Antiseptic Mouthwash and Berry Gum Poultice

This soothing, gum-healing mouthwash protects the soft membranes of the mouth with its astringent, antiseptic, and cell-regenerative ingredients. The gum poultice is used to prevent plaque formation and cleanses the gum between the teeth.

1 teaspoon powdered myrrh

1 teaspoon powdered catechu

½ cup dry white wine

10 drops peppermint essential oil

1 tablespoon fennel seed infusion

1 tablespoon echinacea infusion

See instructions for making herbal infusions on page 36. Place the myrrh, catechu, and dry white wine in a dark-colored glass bottle, secure the lid, and leave it for 1 week to macerate. Shake the bottle daily. Strain through a paper coffee filter, then add the essential oils and infusions. Pour 2 teaspoons of the mouthwash into a cup of mineral water, then swish it around the mouth. Use morning and night.

Caution: Do not use peppermint essential oil if you are taking homeopathic remedies, as this oil is known to interact with many. Talk with your practitioner.

BERRY GUM POULTICE

2 stoned black cherries (mashed)

5 black currants (mashed)

Stir the mashed fruit together. Rub along the gums. Close your mouth for 10 minutes. Chew the fruit thoroughly, then swallow (or spit it out). Rinse with mineral water. For mouth ulcers, chew fresh bilberries, three times a day.

Marshmallow Sunburn Lotion and Fresh Cucumber Poultice

This soothing recipe is for sunburned skin. Marshmallow root has been used for centuries to heal minor skin conditions, including blemishes and allergic rashes.

3 tablespoons dried marshmallow root pieces
2 cups very hot water

Place the marshmallow root in a small bowl and cover with the hot water. Cover and steep overnight (8–10 hours). Strain through a fine mesh and discard the herb. Pour the rich, dark solution into a glass bottle and refrigerate between uses.

Using cotton balls dipped into the lotion, dab lavish amounts over affected areas, then air-dry on the skin.

CUCUMBER POULTICE

½ mashed cucumber
1 tablespoon fresh aloe gel
1 tablespoon marigold leaf infusion (follow instructions for making infusions on page 36)

Place the mashed cucumber in a small bowl, then add the aloe and marigold infusion. Whisk gently. Soak a piece of muslin into the cucumber, aloe, and marigold mixture and set aside. Using a spoon, scoop the rest of the mixture onto the sunburned skin. Place the soaked cloth over the covered skin, making a soothing poultice. Leave for 10 minutes. Remove poultice and allow skin to air-dry. Repeat every 30 minutes, making a fresh poultice each time, until the burning has subsided.

Sage Antibacterial Teeth Granules and Horsetail Gargle

This aromatic tooth powder and gargle has been handed down from generation to generation, long before toothbrushes were invented.

½ teaspoon fresh sage leaves

½ teaspoon lime flowers

½ teaspoon marshmallow leaves

½ teaspoon baking soda

1 teaspoon air-float clay

5 drops spearmint essential oil

Place the ingredients into a small, dark-colored glass jar and shake well.

Dip a clean, damp finger into the granules (some will adhere to your damp skin) and massage your teeth and gums with your fingertip.

HORSETAIL AND ECHINACEA GUM GARGLE

Both herbs are rich in silicon, which heals and strengthens the connective tissue of weak, bleeding gums.

¼ teaspoon (1 ml) echinacea tincture (see instructions for making a tincture on page 35)

2 tablespoons horsetail infusion (see instructions on page 36)

Dilute the echinacea tincture in ¼ cup of mineral water, then add the horsetail infusion. Whisk gently. Lightly brush your gums with a sprinkling of cayenne pepper, then swish your mouth with the gargle.

CONDITION	NATURE'S PANTRY TREATMENT:
Acne	**Use the following remedies for a period of 5–7 days.**

Use the following remedies for a period of 5–7 days.

Drink 1 cup lavender flower infusion upon awakening.

Facial steam of chamomile and yarrow flowers, three times a week.

Rose water and witch hazel facial wash, nightly.

Drink 1 cup sage and yarrow infusion twice daily.

Comfrey, calendula, and chamomile infusion wash.

Fresh cucumber juice applied to acne clusters each night.

Macerated horseradish root in vinegar, wash daily.

½ cup water with 1 tablespoon fresh aloe juice, drink daily.

Eczema

Use these remedies over a period of 5–7 days.

Chickweed infused oil, dabbed daily on lesions.

Burdock root decoction washed over lesions daily.

Plantain leaf and root and sage leaf infusion soak bath.

Chickweed infusion bath, twice daily.

Milk and horseradish root wash, dab itchy skin twice daily.

If covered from head to foot use these remedies twice daily for 7 days.

Apple cider vinegar bath with 5 drops chamomile essential oil.

Strong sage leaf infusion bath, soak for 15 minutes.

Psoriasis

Use these remedies over a period of 1–2 weeks.

Yarrow flower and comfrey root infusion bath, twice weekly.

CONDITION	NATURE'S PANTRY TREATMENT:
Psoriasis (cont'd)	Oatmeal and fresh watercress leaf poultice over lesions. Buttermilk and chamomile essential oil wash, pour into bath daily. Fresh carrot and watercress juice, dabbed on lesions twice daily. Fresh aloe gel and lemon juice, washed over affected skin daily.

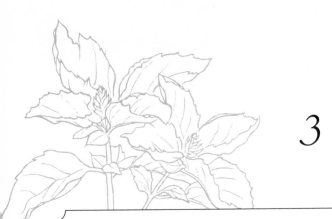

3

Ageless Skin Juices and Shakes

*E*ven the most skillful makeup artist's work is essentially camouflage. There is no substitute for healthy skin, nourished from the inside out. You can make yourself look and feel ageless and beautiful with simple, high-energy raw juices and shakes. Drink your way to beautiful skin with these remarkable cleansing and healing drinks.

Your physical appearance, mental responses, and bodily functions all reflect the way you care for your body, mind, and spirit. So give your body the concentrated micronutrients it needs in the form of raw juices and protein tonics. Both cause physical and biochemical reactions within your body. The following recipes contain combinations of vitamins A, C, and E, and the B complex, as well as antiaging micronutrients silicon, beta-carotene, selenium, potassium, malic acid, calcium, bioflavonoids, bromelin, fluorine, and iron, all of which are easily absorbed in the bloodstream. Acne can be measurably reduced, even to some extent cured, by daily consuming juices rich in the mineral zinc in combination with potent green juices and aloe (such as Ginger and Pepper Clear Skin Juice and Ageless Beautiful Body Skin Food Shake).

Eating the right combination of herbs, fruits, vegetables, and wild edibles will make your hair shine with a vibrant luster, your nails grow stronger and longer, and your eyes sparkle after a few days of incorporating these beautiful skin juices and shakes into your diet. You will look and feel younger.

You are what you eat. Spots, pimples, boils, acne, dull skin, crow's-feet, and puffy eyes are a few telltale signs of skin that's ailing at a cellular level. So make a choice today to change the way you feed your skin. Drink only the best quality, living, liquid nutrition; eat foods that your malnourished skin cells are crying out for. Premature skin aging is not a fact of life. It is the result of unhealthy habits that you can start to change today.

For beautiful, ageless skin, eliminate or consume the following:

Avoid refined or sugar-saturated foods and drinks (especially sodas), salty foods and condiments, fatty and fried foods, and fiber-supplement drinks.

Increase the daily consumption of raw, green, leafy vegetables; herbs and wild edibles; rich fiber foods, including fresh fruit each morning; and whole grains and sprouts.

Drink eight to ten glasses of water daily, skin-nourishing herbal teas, sea vegetable broths, and raw energy juices.

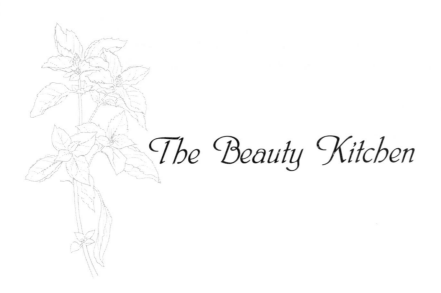

The Beauty Kitchen

Tools of the Trade

You'll need just a few things to get started, many of which you may already own.

A Juicer   This appliance is essential to your beauty kitchen. Before investing in one of the many juicers on the market, see if you can borrow one. That way you can determine which special features you must have or can do without. You might even save money you no longer need to spend on makeup to buy one. My advice is to purchase a versatile juicer, one that can process hard root vegetables, grasses, herbs, leaves, and fruit of all kinds. Keep your own needs in mind; invest in a juicer that will last.

A Large Chopping Board   Avoid wooden chopping boards. These harbor germs and mark easily. The best type of chopping board is tough, resilient, and easy to clean. I prefer a marble slab, but they are rather expensive. Any Formica or polyethylene plastic board will do.

Cutting and Chopping Knives   Good-quality knives for chopping are a must.

Measuring Pitchers   These are essential for measuring yield from various fruits, vegetables, grasses, and herbs. Generally speaking, 1 kg (2.2 pounds) of raw produce will yield approximately 2 cups of fresh juice.

Blender or Food Processor   It is simply not possible to extract juice from low-water-content fruits, such as avocados or bananas. Some fresh produce is considered unjuiceable, which means that the pulp does not easily separate from its water. Simply puree these ingredients with water in a blender or food processor.

Storage Containers   All washed fruit, vegetables, wild edibles, herbs, and grasses to be juiced should be stored in airtight containers in the refrigerator. I use Tupperware, ice cream tubs, and zip-seal plastic bags.

Vegetable Brushes   Most hard-skinned vegetables, fruits, and roots should be scrubbed before juicing. Mud and dirt aren't ingredients in these recipes!

Salad Spinner   All juicing kitchens should have one of these indispensable and inexpensive appliances. Vegetables, leaves, herbs, and grasses need to be crisp so that they can be rolled up into tight balls and juiced effectively.

Strainer   Most juices will need to be strained (even though pulp is harmless and very nutritious). Juices with pulp take more time to digest and assimilate than strained juices. I prefer easy-to-clean stainless steel or dishwasher-safe plastic strainers.

Juicing Your Way to Beautiful Skin

❧ About Drinking the Ageless Beauty Juices and Shakes

These skin-nutrient juice recipes are a form of liquid nutrition, and they require full digestion before entering the stomach. Maximize their healing and nutritious effects; consume them immediately and "chew" thoroughly before swallowing. Sip small mouthfuls, swishing each sip around the mouth several times (just like a mouthwash, but don't spit it out), then swallow. All freshly extracted juices are brightly colored. If they turn a brown color, they are have oxidized and have lost much of their potency. Most of them are meant to be consumed at room temperature on an empty stomach (at least twenty minutes before mealtime). If the juice is to be chilled before consumption, pour it in a glass bottle with crushed ice and let it sit for ten minutes. Strain out the ice before drinking.

Unless otherwise stated, all organic produce can be used in its raw, whole state. Go ahead, put those stems, seeds, cores, skins, or peels right into the juicer. However, commercially grown produce must be peeled, cored, seeded, and have all the stems removed. Do not drink these liquid meals with solid foods. One hour after the juice consumption, drink one twelve-ounce glass of water to flush your system before consuming solid foods, which will ensure full digestion and absorption of the juice nutrients. Save vegetable and herb pulp for composting.

Quantities   The following recipes yield approximately one small glass of juice. However, depending on the actual size of the fresh produce you use, yield will vary. If a recipe recommends drinking a juice more than once a day, you can double or triple the ingredient quantities and make all you'll drink that day at once.

Ageless Hair Juices

Your hair health is a good indication of your general well-being. Each hair shaft taps its nutrients from the papilla, tiny organs that are the hair's powerhouse and that are located within the scalp layers. The following mineral-rich, living juices nourish each individual hair follicle. For a full head of lustrous hair, well-balanced nutrition is an absolute must.

Apple and Celery Growth Promoter Juice

1 tablespoon green pepper juice

¼ cup green apple juice

1 tablespoon cucumber juice

¼ cup celery juice

1 teaspoon parsley juice

Drink one glass of fresh juice twice daily.

Carrot and Cucumber Hair Strength Juice

¼ cup carrot juice

¼ cup cauliflower juice

Drink one glass of juice three times a day.

Carrot and Lettuce Gloss and Glow Juice

1 teaspoon red pepper juice

¼ cup spring carrot juice

1 tablespoon parsley juice

2 tablespoons outer green lettuce leaf juice

Drink one glass of juice three times a day.

Cherry and Pear Silk Wet Look Juice

¼ cup pear juice

¼ cup red cherry juice (remove stones)

Dilute with ½ cup sparkling mineral water and drink daily.

Cucumber and Apricot Shining Glory Juice

3 tablespoons cucumber juice

¼ cup pink apricot juice

Drink one glass three times a day.

Ageless Nail Juices

There is nothing worse than brittle, broken, and flaking nails. You can cover them up with synthetic plastic nails, but that does nothing to strengthen your natural nails underneath. Nails are a structure of complex proteins that derive their nutrients from the white half-moon at the base of each nail, known as the nail matrix. Soft, white nails indicate arthritis. White specks indicate a lack of the mineral zinc in your diet and other dietary changes. Drinking nail-beautifying juices counteracts these deficiencies, feeding the nail essential micronutrients such as silicon, calcium, sulfur, and phosphorus.

Carrot and Parsley Nail Protector Juice

2 tablespoons spring carrot juice

1 tablespoon parsley juice

¼ cup cucumber juice

Drink one glass three times a day.

Cherry and Apricot Strength Shiner Juice

¼ cup red cherry juice

2 tablespoons pink apricot juice

1 tablespoon pear juice

Drink one glass twice daily.

Roots, Leaves, and Florets Length and Strength Juice

2 tablespoons broccoli juice (with the stems)

2 tablespoons green apple juice

1 teaspoon gingerroot juice

3 tablespoons spinach juice (from the dark outer leaves)

Drink one glass daily.

Ageless Eye Juices

The windows to the soul should shine and sparkle. Your eyes can be the focal point of your physical appearance. No amount of makeup can conceal tired, undernourished, or strained eyes. Take good care of your eyes by nourishing them generously with the concentrated micronutrition found in the following juices.

Fennel and Carrot Bright Eyes Juice

2 tablespoons carrot juice

5 tablespoons fennel juice (from bulb and leaves)

Drink one glass diluted with 1 cup water, twice a day.

Strawberry and Mango Sparkling Alive Juice

2 tablespoons ripe mango puree

2 tablespoons ripe strawberry puree

2 tablespoons raspberry puree

½ cup (4 oz.) sparkling mineral water

Drink one chilled glass twice a day.

Cantaloupe and Carrot Sharp Vision Juice

5 tablespoons cantaloupe puree

2 tablespoons carrot juice

Drink one glass three times a day.

Apple and Parsley Eye Shine Bright Juice

¼ cup carrot juice

2 tablespoons green apple juice

1 tablespoon parsley juice

Drink one glass twice a day.

Carrot and Kale Appealing Eyes Juice

½ cup carrot juice

1 tablespoon parsley juice

2 tablespoons kale juice (from the outer leaf)

Drink one glass three times a day.

Apricot and Peach 20–20 Clarity Juice

2 tablespoons pink apricot juice

1 tablespoon peach juice

¼ cup cantaloupe puree

Drink one glass twice a day.

The quality of your skin mirrors your diet. Whatever you feed your body shows up in the condition of your skin. Just like your eyes, your complexion reflects back your general well-being. Pimples and spots spontaneously appear on those days when you are hormonal, depressed, stressed from working too hard, and not taking care of yourself. Thankfully, you can be boost the condition and appearance of your skin by drinking micronutrient-rich, ageless skin juices. These juices are high in the vitamins A, C, E, and B_{12} with the minerals selenium, beta-carotene, potassium, silicon, and iron. So go ahead, drink your way to beautiful skin.

Strawberry and Cherry Age Wonder Juice

1 tablespoon carrot juice

2 tablespoons apple juice

¼ cup red cherry juice

½ cup sparkling mineral water (chilled)

Drink one glass twice daily.

Lettuce and Pear Wrinkle-Smoothing Juice

1 tablespoon carrot juice

1 tablespoon parsley juice

¼ cup kale (from the outer leaf) juice

1 tablespoon pear juice

Drink one glass twice a day.

Asparagus and Beet Root Soft-Touch Juice

1 tablespoon carrot juice

2 teaspoons parsley juice

3 tablespoons lettuce leaves (from the outer green leaves)

2 tablespoons pear juice

Drink one glass three times a day.

Ginger and Pepper Clear Skin Juice

¼ cup carrot juice

2 teaspoons fresh gingerroot juice

1 tablespoon green pepper juice

1 tablespoon cabbage (from the outer leaf) juice

½ cup apple juice

Drink one glass daily.

Grape and Apricot Youthful Look Juice

1 tablespoon red-orange mango puree

1 tablespoon passion fruit juice

1 tablespoon pink apricot puree

¼ cup red grape juice

Drink one glass twice a day.

Spinach and Carrot Clear Complexion Juice

¼ cup carrot juice

1 tablespoon kale (from the outer leaf) juice

1 tablespoon spinach (from the outer leaf) juice

3 tablespoons pear juice

Drink one glass twice a day.

Cantaloupe and Peach Silky Soft-Touch Juice

2 tablespoons peach juice

2 tablespoons kiwi juice

4 tablespoons cantaloupe juice

Drink one glass daily.

Squash and Parsley Radiant Alive Juice

1 tablespoon peach juice

1 tablespoon celery (stick and leaf) juice

2 teaspoons parsley juice

1 tablespoon green squash juice

2 tablespoons watercress juice

Drink one glass twice a day.

Beautiful Face, Beautiful Body

❧ *Lime and Grapefruit Skin Zest Juice*

1 tablespoon (sweet, juicy) orange juice

1 tablespoon lime juice

4 tablespoons pink grapefruit juice

Peel rind off these citrus fruits before juicing, leaving pith. Drink one glass three times a day.

❧ *Strawberry and Watermelon Summer Fresh Juice*

2 tablespoons ripe strawberry puree

5 tablespoons watermelon puree

½ cup sparkling mineral water

Drink one chilled glass twice daily.

❧ *Ageless Appeal Juices*

Certain whole foods have well-established reputations as aphrodisiacs. For instance, the ancient Egyptian's government banned the consumption of onions because they were thought to drive men wild with passion. There are many fruits, vegetables, herbs, and spices whose biochemical makeup creates a similar effect. The French have known for centuries the power of unpretentious celery. Recent research confirms that celery does, in fact, contain pheromones. Fennel's reputation as a sex enhancer dates back to Roman times. The rich, sexy, micronutrients in these following juice recipes will nurture your beautiful body and hopefully lead to a happy hour between the sheets.

Fennel and Apricot Love Nectar Appeal Juice

¼ cup pineapple juice

1 tablespoon pink apricot puree

2 teaspoons ripe mango puree

2 teaspoons fennel juice (from the bulb and leaves)

Drink one glass three times a day.

Strawberry and Cherry Fruit Zinger Juice

¼ cup ripe strawberry puree

¼ cup red cherry juice

1 teaspoon rose hip juice

Drink one glass three times a day.

Rose Hip and Black Currant Screwdriver Sexy Juice

2 tablespoons blood orange juice

1 tablespoon rose hip juice

5 tablespoons black currant juice

Peel the orange before juicing, leaving the pith on the fruit. Drink one glass three times a day.

Carrot and Fennel Aphrodite Juice

1 tablespoon carrot juice

1 tablespoon kale juice (from the outer green leaves)

2 teaspoons onion juice

1 tablespoon apple juice

2 tablespoons fennel juice

Drink one glass three times a day.

Grape and Peach Love Potion Juice

¼ cup red grape juice

¼ cup peach juice

Drink one glass three times a day.

Your skin essentially consists of water and about 25 percent protein. Protein is the vital component that holds the skin together. Collagen is a protein. Elastin is a protein. Hormones and enzymes are proteins. Your skin is your body's protective guard that not only gives you form and structure, it keeps out germs, bacteria, and some viruses. You need to replenish skin proteins daily as your body only manufactures fourteen of the twenty-two it requires. Your body gets the missing eight amino acids from your diet. The following recipes are replete with essential nutrients and other necessary skin foods. These concentrated liquid meals also will counteract skin-damaging agents that affect the quality and appearance of your living suit.

≈ *Ageless Beautiful Face Morning Cocktail*

1 teaspoon dandelion leaf juice

1 teaspoon lecithin granules

2 teaspoons dill juice

2 small apples

½ banana

5 ripe strawberries

2 teaspoons blackstrap molasses

3 tablespoons live-culture plain yogurt

½ cup buttermilk

1 teaspoon brewer's yeast

Puree prepared produce for 30 seconds on a high speed, then 30 seconds on a low speed. If you are unable to juice fresh herbs, dilute ¼ teaspoon of the powdered herb (dandelion and dill, which can be purchased from health food stores), in 2 teaspoons of water. Pour cocktail into a chilled glass and drink each morning before breakfast.

Ageless Beautiful Body Skin Food Shake

1-inch slice watermelon, with seeds

½ teaspoon powdered brewer's yeast

½ teaspoon powdered spirulina

½ teaspoon powdered propolis

½ teaspoon powdered royal jelly

1 teaspoon fresh aloe juice

1 teaspoon ginseng root juice

8 oz. red grapes

10 ripe strawberries or 4 pink apricots

2 teaspoons blossom honey

Chop the melon into small chunks. Puree all the ingredients in a blender or food processor for 30 seconds on a high speed, then 30 seconds on a low speed. Pour into a chilled glass and drink once a day.

Ageless Facial Skin-Food Shake

30 young dandelion leaves

½ fennel bulb

10 small apples

8 oz. green grapes

1 tablespoon barley grass juice

2 teaspoons pure maple syrup (grade A)

½ teaspoon powdered spirulina

1 teaspoon powdered royal jelly

1 teaspoon powdered propolis

1 teaspoon fresh aloe juice

½ cup fresh coconut milk

2 teaspoons live-culture plain yogurt

Process the dandelion, fennel, apples, grapes, and barley grass in the juicer. Strain, then add to the other ingredients in the blender. If you are unable to obtain fresh coconut milk, use ½ cup of fresh coconut meat and blend with 2 cups of water, then strain. Blend for 30 seconds on high, then 30 seconds on low. Drink at room temperature once a day.

Green Protein Potency Shake

1 teaspoon fresh wheat grass juice

2 teaspoons fresh aloe juice

2 tablespoons fresh dandelion leaf juice

2 tablespoons alfalfa sprout juice (from 6 days' growth)

1 teaspoon parsley juice

¼ cup apple juice

2 teaspoons powdered spirulina

¼ cup soy sprout juice (from 4 days' growth)

1 cup green grape juice

Process ingredients in blender, 30 seconds on a high speed, then 30 seconds on low speed. Drink at room temperature twice a day.

Beautiful Face, Beautiful Body

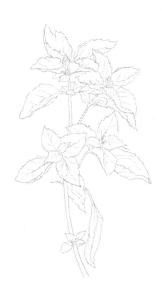

Appendix

Weights and Measures

⅛ teaspoon = 0.5 ml

¼ teaspoon = 1 ml

½ teaspoon = 2 ml

1 teaspoon = 5 ml

3 teaspoons = 1 tablespoon (15 ml)

4 tablespoons = ¼ cup (60 ml)

8 tablespoons = ½ cup (120 ml)

12 tablespoons = ¾ cup (178 ml)

16 tablespoons = 1 cup (240 ml)

¼ liter = 8 oz., 1 cup, ½ pint

½ liter = 16 oz., 2 cups, 1 pint

1 liter = 32 oz., 4 cups, 1 quart

2 liters = 64 oz., 8 cups, 2 quarts

4 liters = 128 oz., 4 quarts, 1 gallon

Juice of one apple = 2 tablespoons

Juice of one lemon = 3 tablespoons

Juice of one orange = 5 tablespoons

Juice of one grapefruit = ½ cup

Bach Flower Remedies
Edward Bach Centre
Mt. Vernon, Bidwell,
   Wallingford
Oxon OX10 OPZ England

Aroma Vera
PO Box 399
Weaverville, CA 96093
Tel:(800) 437-3301
(100 percent pure
   essential oils)

Aphrodite
282 Bleecker Street
New York, NY 10014
Tel:(212) 989-6440
(Additive-free clays, oils,
   herbs, spices)

Indiana Botanic Garden
   Inc.
3401 West Thirty-seventh
   Ave.
Hobart, IN 46342
Tel:(219) 974-4040
(Resins, herbal tinctures)

Natives Herb Co.
1010 Forty-second Street
Philadelphia, PA 19123
Tel:(215) 601-0702
(Organic herbs, essential
   oils, base oils)

Artisa Industries Inc.
1082 Post Road
Darien, CT 06820
Tel:(203) 655-0881
(Cold-pressed oils)

Brushy Mountain Bee
   Farm
610 Bethany Church Road
Morvian Falls, NC 28654
Tel:(800) 233-7929;
   Fax:(910) 921-2681
(Honey, bee pollen,
   beeswax)

Once Upon a Thyme
3606 State Route 22
85 Battenkill Evergreens
Salem, NY 12865
Tel:(518) 854-7924
(Live herb plants, catalog
   on request)

American Association of
   Holistic Healing Cen-
   ters
109 Holly Crescent, Suite
   201
Virginia Beach, VA 23451
Tel:(804) 422-9033

The Essential Oil Com-
   pany
PO Box 206
Lake Oswego, OR 97034
Tel:(800) 729-5912
(Aromatherapy supplies)

Avena Botanicals
20 Mill Street
Rockland, NE 04841
(207) 574-0694
(Organic herbs and essen-
   tial oils, catalogue $2)

Lavender Lane
7337 Roseville Road
Sacramento, CA 95842
Tel:(888) 593-4400;
   Fax:(916) 339-0842

Internet: http://
www.choicemail.com/
lavenderln/
(Selections of bottles and
storage jars)

Penn Herb Co.
603 North Second Street
Philadelphia, PA 19123
Tel:(800) 523-9971
(Almost every herb you
will ever need)

Ginghams's Spice Ltd.
Nancy Booth
PO Box 88 pcs
Gardenville, PA 18926
Tel:(215) 348-8021;
Fax:(215) 348-8021
(Glycerin, rose and orange
flower water, red turkey
oil, vanilla bean, essen-
tial oils)

Frontier Co-op Herbs
3021 78th Street, PO Box
299
Norway, IA 52318
Tel:(800) 669-3275;
Fax:(800) 717-4372
Internet: http://www.
frontier herb.com
(Free catalog)

Magazines and Periodicals

The Herb Quarterly
PO Box 689
San Anselmo, CA 94960
Tel:(415) 455-9540

Vegetarian Times
PO Box 570
Oak Park, IL 60303
Tel:(708) 848-8100

Soap Cosmetics Chemicals
Specialties
446 Broad Hollow Road
Melville, NY 11747

Cosmetics & Toiletries
Box 318
Wheaton, IL 60189

Skin Inc.
Box 318
Wheaton, IL 60189

Drug & Cosmetic Industry
747 Third Avenue
New York, NY 10017

The Herbal Connection
PO Box 245
Silver Springs, PA 17571

HerbalGram
PO Box 201660
Austin, TX 78720

Acacia Vera
Common/folk name: gum arabic, Egyptian thorn

Almond (prunus amygdalus)
Common name: sweet almond

Aloes (aloe spicata)
Common name: aloe vera, the "burn" plant

Anise (pimpinella anisum)
Common name: aniseed

Argrimony (agrimonia eupatoria)
Common/folk name: cockleburr, sticklewort

Balm of Lemon (melissa officinalis)
Common name: lemon balm

Bay (laurus nobilis)

Basil (ocimum basilicum)

Benzoin (styrax benzoin)

Bergamot (citrus bergamia)

Bilberry (vaccinium myrtillus)

Blackberry (rubus fruticosus)

Black Currant (ribes nigrum)

Burdock (articium lappa)
Japanese name: gobo

Calendula (calendula officinalis)
Herbal/folklore name: herbal sunshine

Catnip (nepeta cataria)
Common name: cat mint

Catechu (acacia catechu)
Herbal folklore names: cutch, terra japonica, gambir

Celery (apium graveolens)

Chamomile (chamomilla matricaria)
Herbal/folklore name: baby remedy plant

Chickweed (stellaria media)

Cinnamon (cinnamonum zeylanicum)

Cleavers (galium aparine)
Herbal/folklore name: goose grass, bed straw, catchweed, our lady's bedstraw

Clover (Red—trifolum pratense, White—trifolium repens)

Cloves (syzygium aromaticum)

Comfrey (symphytum officinale)
Herbal/folklore name: burn healing plant

Cornflower (centaurea cyanus)
Herbal/folklore name: bachelor's button

Dandelion (taraxacum officinale)
Common names: lion's tooth, piss-in-bed, wild endive, blowball

Dill (anethum graveolens)
Common name: colic remedy herb

Echinacea Root (echinacea augustifolia)
Herbal/folklore names: comb flower, red sunflower, root coneflower

Elderflower (sambucus nigra)
Herbal/folklore names: elder mother plant, fairy tree, fever berry

Elecampane (inula helenium)

Eucalyptus (eucalyptus globulus)

Evening Primrose (oenothera biennis)

Eyebright (euphrasis officinale)

Fennel (foeniculum officinale/vulgare)

Feverfew (pyrethrum parthenium)
  Medicinal folklore name: women's herb

Garlic (allium sativum)
  Medicinal folklore name: antimicrobial
  herb

Geranium (pelargonium odorantissimun)
  Common name: sweet geranium

Ginger (zingiber officinale)

Goldenseal (hydrastis canadensis)
  Herbal/folklore names: yaller root,
  goldthread, yellow puccoon, ground
  raspberry

Hisbiscus (hibiscus rosa-sineursis)

Horsetail (equisetum arvensis)
  Medicinal folklore names: mane's tail,
  shave grass, pewterwort, bottle brush

Hyssop (hyssopus officinale)

Ivy (ampelopsis quinquefolia)
  Herbal/folklore names: woodbine, Virginia creeper, five leaves, false grape

Juniper (juniperus communis)

Lavender (lavandula angustifolia)

Lemon Verbena (aloysia triphylla)

Linden Flowers (tilia europea)

Linseed (linum usitissimum)

Licorice (glyceyrrhiza flabra)

Lobelia (lobella inflata)
  Herbal/folklore name: Indian
  tobacco

Marigold (see calendula)

Marjoram (origanum majorana)
  Common name: Sweet majoram

Marshmallow (althaea officinalis)

Mullein (verbasum thapsus)
  Medicinal folklore name: Quaker rouge

Mustard (brassica niga)

Myrrh (commiphora myrrha)

Nasturtium (tropaeolum majus)

Nettles: (urtica urens)
  Common name: great stinging nettle

Nutmeg (myristicza fragrans)

Oats (avena sativa)

Onion (allium cepa)

Orange flower (citrus auranthium)

Parsley (petrolselinum crispum)

Pennyroyal (mentha pulequin)
  Herbal/folklore names: tickweed,
  squawmint

Peppermint (mentha piperita)

Plantain (plantago major)
  Medicinal folklore name: ribwort

Potato (solanum tuberosum)
  Common name: earth tubers

Prickly Ash (zanthoxylum americanum)
  Medicinal folklore names: yellow
  wood, toothache bush

Primrose (primula orleracnum)

Rhubarb (rheum palmatum)

Rose, red (rosa gallica)

Rose Hip (rosa cinina)

Rosemary (rosmarinus officinalis)

Sage (salvia officinalis)
  Common name: garden sage

St.-John's-wort (hypericium perforatum)
Herbal/folklore names: flower of the fairies, wolf medicine

Sarsaparilla (simlax officinalis)

Soap Wort (saponaria officinalis)
Medicinal folklore name: bouncing bet

Tansy (tanacetum vulgare)

Tea Tree (melanlenca alternifolia)

Thyme (thymus vulgaris)

Tobacco (nicotiana tabacum)
Common name: Smoke weed

Violet (viola odorata)

Walnut (juglans regia)
Herbal/folklore names: butternut, oil nut

Watercress (nasturtium officinale)

Wheat Grass (triticum aestivum)

Wintergreen (gaultheria procumbens)
Common name: Canadian tea

Witch Hazel (hamamelis virginana)
Herbal/folklore names: winter bloom, snapping hazel, spotted alder

Yarrow (achillea millefolium)
Medicinal folklore name: squirrel tail

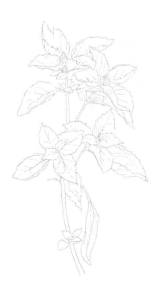

Index

Nail care, 133
Nail juices
    Length strength, 213
    Nail protector, 212
    Strength shiner, 213
Nasturtium (botanical name), 229
Nasturtium rinse, 166
Natural hair dyes, 162
Nettle (botanical name), 229
Nettle rinse, 150
Nutmeg (botanical name), 229

Oatmeal, 23
Oils
    Cold-pressed, 11–12
    Infused oils, 8–11
    Macerated oils, 38
    Pure essential oils, 7–11
Oily hair treatments, 151
Olive oil, 11
Olive's lightening paste
    and mullein rinse, 167
Orange flower (botanical name), 229
Orange flower refresher, 67
Orange-lavender mist, 68
Orange flower moisturizing oil, 129
Orrisroot, 23

Palm and ball washing granules, 143
Pamela's hibiscus (hair coloring) rinse, 164
Papain, 23
Parsley (botanical name), 229
Patch skin test, 34
Patricia's acne sage pack, 100
Patsy's spot eliminator formula, 192
Peach, 18
Pectin, 23
Peppermint (botanical name), 229
Petula's antidandruff rinse, 154
Ph tests, 154
Plantain, 16
Plantain skin mist, 69
Plantain skin wash, 195

Pore-tight mask, 51
Powders
    Body, 117
    Dusting, 93
    Feet, 137
Prepaste color stay infusion, 173
Primrose, 229
Propolis, 23
    Chapped lip salve, 190
Protein shake, 224
Pumice, 24
Purchasing
    Herbs, 12–17
    Natural resources, 17–25
    Oils, 7–11
Purifying body-balance seaweed bath, 118

Queenie's honey-barley mask, 53

Raspberries, 38
Reggie's raw potato compress, 179
Relaxing herbal massage oil, 126
Rhassoul mud, 24
Rhubarb (botanical name), 229
Rhubarb highlight paste, 171
Richly moisturizing mask, 54
Rinses
    Colorants, 161
    Hair, 148
    Nourishing skin, 85
Rose (botanical name), 229
Rose hip (botanical name), 229
Rose hip facial mist (see Josephine's linseed
    moisturizer), 62
Rose hip–comfrey mist, 63
Rose hip–chamomile mist, 64
Rosemary (botanical name), 229
Rosemary-walnut (hair blackening) paste,
    165
Rose-scented moisturizing skin splash, 83
Rosewater
    Bath, 111
    Cleanser, 74

For the natural beauty beginner: To ensure an easy transition into the exciting world of natural beauty, I have put together some bathing and hair dye starter kits, which include a rich variety of herbal, homeopathic, and aromatherapy ingredients, with color and gem energy therapies that are especially designed for your inside-outside optimum skin health, ageless cellular beauty and spiritual healing.

- *Marigold & Mullein Highlighter Kit*
- *Skin-renewal Bathing Kit*
- *Women's Healing Bath Kit*
- *Amethyst & Lavender Bathing Meditation Kit*
- *Wrinkle-away Bathing Mask Kit*
- *Nasturtium & Walnut "Gray-away" Dye Kit*
- *Cellulite-away Massage, Bath & Tea Kit*
- *Aromatherapy "Weight-Loss" Bath Kit*
- *Burdock, Henna & Safflower "Auburn Tint" Kit*
- *Stress Reduction Bath Kit*

Each kit yields two baths or treatments. These all-natural, cruelty-free, and organic treatments are packaged in recycled material. To order call:
Jaqulene Roth: (704) 871-1765 or E-mail: rothbeauty@Mailcity.com

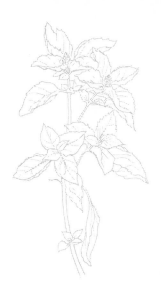

About the Author

Jaqulene Harper-Roth, a qualified holistic nutritionist, nature care therapist, and home-practicing herbalist, studied at The School of Natural Healing and Nutritional Medicine, Sussex, England. She has spent the past ten years researching and experimenting with the cruelty-free, alternative cosmetics and whole-body remedies found in this book. As a nutritional correction therapist in England, she began making, prescribing, and demonstrating how to use natural ingredients to promote inner health and outer beauty. She was her own guinea pig for all the remedies, cosmetics, juices, and shakes in this book. She admits that although most of her experiences have been educational and enjoyable, experimenting with hair dyes resulted in some astonishing hues. She now lives with her husband, three children, and their twelve cats in their pleasant, peaceful home in North Carolina.